Great Health Care

J. Timothy Harrington · Eric D. Newman
Editors

Great Health Care

Making It Happen

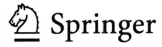 Springer

Editors
J. Timothy Harrington, MD
Division of Rheumatology
School of Medicine and Public Health
University of Wisconsin
Madison, WI, USA
timharrington@charter.net

Eric D. Newman, MD
Department of Rheumatology
Clinical Innovations
Division of Medicine
Geisinger Health System
Danville, PA, USA
arthman@aol.com

ISBN 978-1-4614-1197-0   e-ISBN 978-1-4614-1198-7
DOI 10.1007/978-1-4614-1198-7
Springer New York Dordrecht Heidelberg London

Library of Congress Control Number: 2011940809

Printed on acid-free paper

Springer is part of Springer Science+Business Media (www.springer.com)

Prologue: Sooner or Later We Are all Patients

Blame my parents. When I was 8 years old, they bought me a seemingly innocuous poster for my room – three turtles traveling down a river. The first turtle was paddling furiously, the second turtle was paddling furiously, but the third turtle had climbed out of its shell, had flipped the shell over, was sitting in it, and was using two oars to effortlessly navigate the river. The title of the poster read … "there's always a better way"

Eric Newman

I have always questioned the status quo. On an October night in the mid-1960s, a 52-year-old man was transported to the emergency room of the Massachusetts General Hospital with acute chest pain. His heart stopped twice, and he was twice resuscitated. As the intern on-call, I was expected to admit him to an unoccupied bed on the private service ward that did not have a cardiac care unit yet. In that room, I was convinced, my patient would die that night.

So I called a surgery intern friend and "borrowed" a bed for my patient in the fully equipped surgical recovery room, where he survived two more arrhythmias. The following morning, the Chief of Surgery objected to this "medical" patient using a "surgical" bed. The Chief of Medicine supported my decision, and the Mass General soon established a cardiac care unit for its private service

Tim Harrington

Health Care Will not Reform Itself

George C. Halvorson, Chief Executive Officer, Kaiser Permanente

Great Health Care is written for all of us. Sooner or later our loved ones and we will all be patients and will desire the care described in this book. Being a physician or a health insurance executive doesn't come with a "get out of jail free" card. We all need to know what great care looks like and how it works – to be informed consumers and active participants in achieving it.

This book is written by a collection of physicians and nurses who are dedicated to building great healthcare programs within their own practices and health systems, and feel it is important to share these ideas in these challenging times when healthcare reform needs to move from abstract policy to reality.

There are two parts of providing healthcare – knowledge and process. Knowledge guides what care should be delivered, and process determines how it is delivered. There are many publications for the public and physicians about what should be done for every human ailment, but very few about how health care can best be provided in practices and local health systems to those who need it, dependably and at the lowest possible cost. Our recent national healthcare debate has helped make the issues more public. Now we need to define and implement the positive changes that will transform how health care is delivered – best quality at an affordable cost.

This book is for all who are ready to help improve how health care is provided – the public, patients, and the healthcare media who have the unique power to change thinking broadly; those who determine health policy and financing; and physicians motivated to change. Without knowing how better health care works, how can we know what to ask for, and how we can work together to make things better? Collins and Porras wrote a book about what makes businesses great. These organizations create BHAG's for themselves – Big Hairy Audacious Goals. Well, this book is our BHAG, and we believe this is what it's going to take for us to pull our health system out of its nose-dive. It is not for the squeamish, the faint-of-heart, those who claim we already have "the greatest health care in the World", or those who wish to maintain or just tweak the status quo within which they are personally advantaged.

Great Health Care focuses on improving care for chronic diseases. It is these chronic diseases – heart and vascular conditions, obesity, asthma, arthritis, osteoporosis, diabetes, and chronic kidney disease, alone and in combination, for which the greatest quality gaps exist between what care is best and how effectively it is provided. They wear people down, compromise the quality and productivity of life, and eventually contribute to premature disability and death. They account for 75% of US healthcare costs. For this reason, patients with chronic diseases are the targets of cost-reducing strategies by the health insurance industry, like preexisting conditions and pre-certifications. We have also included a chapter on end-of-life care alternatives that we view as essential to our purpose. The complexity of caring for chronic diseases across time, involving multiple medical specialties and repeated episodes of care, provides the greatest challenge for both healthcare providers and patients, and for improving our Nation's health and our economy.

The editors and contributors to *Great Health Care* are highly interested in optimizing delivery of care processes. We are drawn to understanding how things work and making them better. Most of us have been this way all our lives. We probably think more like engineers. We use both process management methods developed in many other industries to design and implement better ways of doing things, and also research methods when they fit the need. Our shared perspectives have drawn us to one another. We are convinced that it is not only what we know, but also how effectively we work with others in healthcare teams, that makes all the difference.

We will begin by providing a perspective on why health care is what it is and how this needs to change. We will then share our stories about great care, and describe the different perspectives and quality improvement processes that are critical for designing and providing great care for chronic diseases. Finally, we will discuss the controversies that are confusing and delaying these necessary improvements.

Great Health Care is within our reach whether we are on the providing or receiving end. We hope you will join us on our quest!

Contents

Contributors

Martin J. Abrahamson, MD, FACP Joslin Diabetes Center,
Harvard Medical School, Boston, MA, USA

Richard S. Beaser, MD Joslin Diabetes Center, Harvard Medical School,
Boston, MA, USA

Stacy Brethauer, MD Bariatric and Metabolic Institute, The Cleveland Clinic,
Cleveland, OH, USA

Julie Brown, CCMEP Joslin Diabetes Center, Harvard Medical School,
Boston, MA, USA

Karen Cooper, DO Bariatric and Metabolic Institute, The Cleveland Clinic,
Cleveland, OH, USA

John J. Cush, MD Baylor University Medical Center, Dallas, TX, USA

Richard M. Dell, MD Department of Orthopedics, Kaiser Permanente,
Downey, CA, USA

Mark D. Faber Division of Nephrology, Henry Ford Hospital, Detroit, MI, USA

Kathi Farrell, RN, BSN, PHN Marian Medical Center, Catholic HealthCare West,
Santa Maria, CA, USA

Michael B. Foggs, MD Allergy/Immunology. Advocate Health Care,
Chicago, IL, USA

J. Timothy Harrington, MD Division of Rheumatology, University of Wisconsin
School of Medicine and Public Health, Madison, WI, USA

Sangeeta Kashyap, MD Bariatric and Metabolic Institute, The Cleveland Clinic,
Cleveland, OH, USA

Richard D. Lueker, MD New Heart Center for Wellness, Fitness,
and Cardiac Rehabilitation, Albuquerque, NM, USA

Beth A. McCormick, MS New Heart Center for Wellness, Fitness, and Cardiac Rehabilitation, Albuquerque, NM, USA

Eric D. Newman, MD Department of Rheumatology, Clinical Innovations, Division of Medicine, Geisinger Health System, Danville, PA, USA

Jo-Anne M. Rizzotto, MEd, RD, LDN, CDE Joslin Diabetes Center, Harvard Medical School, Boston, MA, USA

Philip Schauer, MD Bariatric and Metabolic Institute, The Cleveland Clinic, Cleveland, OH, USA

Kenneth Snow, MD Joslin Diabetes Center, Harvard Medical School, Boston, MA, USA

Sandeep S. Soman, MD Division of Nephrology, Henry Ford Hospital, Detroit, MI, USA

Kathleen Sullivan, RN, MSN Marian Medical Center, Catholic Health Care West, Santa Maria, CA, USA

Martha L. Twaddle, MD Midwest Palliative and Hospice Care Center, Glenview, IL, USA

Jerry Yee, MD Division of Nephrology, Henry Ford Hospital, Detroit, MI, USA

Part I
Caring for Chronic Diseases: How We Got into This Mess, and Why We Need to Get Out of It

J. Timothy Harrington

> *Now, in a time of both promising and fearful transformation of health care, the profession of medicine must... ask how we will get better at what we must accomplish together if we are to accomplish it at all*
>
> *(Terry Clemmer MD, Vicki Spuhler RN, Donald Berwick MD, MPP, and Thomas Nolan, PhD [1]).*

Redesigning health care, and that for chronic diseases in particular, is the focus of our book for two simple reasons.

First: the current system is broken. It costs too much, and too often yields little value for patients and society.

Second: it's fixable. We're convinced of that. Transforming chronic disease care into processes that produce better outcomes at reduced cost is no pipe dream. More than a few examples of such achievements are out there and not just for individuals, but for whole populations treated in exceptional programs. What's missing is the will to adopt and duplicate these models all across our country.

Part I will explore the evolution of the United States health system over the last half century and the root causes of its current shortcomings. I rely on a broad range of information and writings, but also draw from my own experiences in a career that has spanned this same piece of time. A variety of professional experiences in multiple health care environments – plus an interest in organizations and how they work – adds up to one physician's struggle to adapt to rapid changes and the growing chaos that has enveloped us all.

J.T. Harrington, MD
Division of Rheumatology, University of Wisconsin School of Medicine
and Public Health, Madison, WI, USA

And finally, how great health care is beginning to emerge – a "run to daylight" in Vince Lombardi's words.

Reference

1. Clemmer TP, Spuhler VJ, Berwick DM, Nolan TW. Cooperation: the foundation of improvement. Ann Intern Med. 1998;128:1004–9.

Chapter 1
Why Chronic Diseases?

J. Timothy Harrington

Keywords Chronic disease • Redesign • Health care delivery • Cost • Ineffective treatment • Opportunity • Improvement

> *Where's the beef?*
>
> Clara Peller, Wendy's Commercial, 1984

> *A hard-driving, hard-living attorney friend called me one day in 1975 when we were both in our mid-30's. "Tim, I watched this TV show last night about the 8 risk factors for an early heart attack. I'd have all 8, except I stopped smoking again last weekend! My Dad died of a heart attack at 45. What should I do?"*
>
> *"Ray, I've got just the guy for you," I replied. So Ray saw my hard-driving preventive cardiologist colleague, and Myron told him, "Ray, don't come back to see me till you do everything I tell you, because if you don't change your ways, you won't live much longer, and it will be bad for my reputation."*
>
> *Ray called me back – "I'll show that guy!"*
>
> *He did everything Myron told him to do. Quit smoking for good that day, began walking, and then running every noon at the Y. He switched to a Mediterranean diet and began meditating to reduce his stress. Eight months later, back he goes to Myron, 70 pounds lighter with a normal blood pressure, a resting pulse of 65, and a low cholesterol. Myron said, "I never thought I'd see you again."*
>
> *But Ray had drunk the Kool-Aid; he was just getting started. Next he organized a running group, and finished a marathon 2 years later. He quit his high stress law practice, bought a video store franchise with his son, and they made a lot of money. He is still going strong at 70*
>
> J. Timothy Harrington

J.T. Harrington, MD (✉)
Division of Rheumatology, University of Wisconsin School of Medicine
and Public Health, Madison, WI, USA
e-mail: timharrington@charter.net

J.T. Harrington and E.D. Newman (eds.), *Great Health Care: Making It Happen*,
DOI 10.1007/978-1-4614-1198-7_1, © Springer Science+Business Media, LLC 2012

3

"What do I have to do?"
"It's hard to summarize, but there are three things." Did you
ever notice how there are always three things? *"Three things,"*
he says. *"Exercise. Nutrition. And commitment."*
"The biggest one – and the biggest change for most people – is
exercise. It's the secret to great health."
A conversation between Chris Crowley and Henry S. Lodge
MD, the patient and the physician, authors of Younger Next
Year.
My doctor recently told me that jogging could add years to my
life. I think he was right. I feel ten years older already.

Milton Berle

Raise your hand and count yourself lucky if you've made it through middle age
without knowing someone who's been knocked down by complications of (to name
a few) obesity, arthritis, asthma, or heart disease. Tens of millions of Americans
suffer from one or more of the chronic diseases listed in Table 1.1. They are common and they are deadly, as Table 1.2 illustrates. In contrast to acute illnesses and
injuries, they require the attention of multiple providers for years or decades.
Collectively, chronic diseases consumed 75% of the $2.3 trillion US healthcare bud-
get in 2008, according to the Centers for Medicare and Medicaid Services and the
Centers for Disease Control and Prevention.

Table 1.1 Prevalence of common chronic diseases in the United States across all ages[a] [1]

Hypertension	33.9%
Cholesterol disorders	20.9%
Respiratory diseases	20.0%
Arthritis	15.8%
Heart disease	12.5%
Diabetes	12.3%
Eye disorders	11.1%
Asthma	10.7%
Chronic respiratory infections	8.8%

[a] Twenty-three percent of Americans have one chronic condition, and 26% have more than one

Table 1.2 Chronic diseases are the leading causes of death among US adults of age 65 and over [2]

Heart disease	32.4%
Cancer	21.7%
Stroke	8.0%
Chronic lung diseases	5.9%
Influenza and pneumonia	3.1%
Diabetes	3.0%
Alzheimer's disease	3.0%
All other causes	22.8%

Source: CDC, National Center for Health Statistics, National Vital Statistics Report (2002)

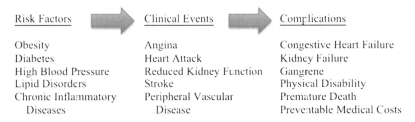

Risk Factors	Clinical Events	Complications
Obesity	Angina	Congestive Heart Failure
Diabetes	Heart Attack	Kidney Failure
High Blood Pressure	Reduced Kidney Function	Gangrene
Lipid Disorders	Stroke	Physical Disability
Chronic Inflammatory	Peripheral Vascular	Premature Death
Diseases	Disease	Preventable Medical Costs

Fig. 1.1   The life history of atherosclerosis

Is our society getting high value for its healthcare dollar? Sadly, the answer is No [3]. Less than half of the people with any chronic disease are being diagnosed and treated early and well. Improvements eked out through the years have been incremental and spotty. Whether you live or die should not depend on who you know or how close you live to an excellent clinic or who is staffing the emergency room. Risk factors like obesity, environmental toxins, and stress that bring on and worsen chronic diseases are actually increasing, and smoking continues to cause heart and lung disease, and cancers. Perhaps the most tragic and threadbare hole in our safety net is positioned directly under children living in poverty, for they are the ones experiencing alarmingly high frequencies of obesity and severe asthma.

If these diseases are not interrupted, they erode the patient's quality of life, and that of his or her loved ones. They remove productive people from their careers and jobs and cause economic and emotional ruin. In their advanced stages, the costs of treatment are astronomical and often futile. Witness that 27% of Medicare dollars are spent during the last year of peoples' lives, often for expensive intensive care in an era when palliative and hospice care alternatives are available and preferred by many, but are underutilized and undersupported.

We already have the knowledge and tools to reduce the impact of most chronic diseases through prevention and early intervention. Let's look at two examples: atherosclerosis and rheumatoid arthritis.

Atherosclerosis is a degenerative disease that replaces healthy arterial walls with inflammatory cholesterol plaques (Fig. 1.1). The clues to a person's risk for atherosclerosis can be plucked right from their family history of heart attacks, strokes, kidney failure, and poor circulation. It's a well-recognized continuum. We know that untreated atherosclerosis will lead first to heart attacks and stroke, and then heart failure, disability, and death. But we also know there are red flags – predisposing conditions – that wave starkly on the horizon decades in advance of a person's arteries becoming clogged and fragile. Many years in which to intervene! These are obesity, high blood pressure and cholesterol, and diabetes. In every case, from education to medication, we physicians know what to do. We can reduce these risks and/or prevent clinical events through early diagnosis and treatment. We can even slow and reverse atherosclerosis through secondary prevention following early clinical events and through more effective management of patients with late disease.

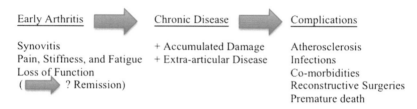

Fig. 1.2 The life history of rheumatoid arthritis

Let's move to the second example of rheumatoid arthritis (RA), a chronic disease close to the editors' hearts because we are both rheumatologists. My own grand-mother and mother were disabled by RA and died early due to complications of the less effective treatments available to their generations. Rheumatoid arthritis pre-dominately affects women in their middle years, and early in my career, treatments seldom provided either relief or disease control. Then medical researchers began to understand why the joint linings and other tissues become inflamed in these patients. They also recognized that they generally died a decade earlier than others because of the corrosive effects of chronic inflammation not only on the joints, but also on the arteries. Inflammatory chemicals circulating through the body cause premature atherosclerosis leading to heart attacks and strokes – yet another risk factor for ath-erosclerosis (Fig. 1.2). Inflammation also robs strength from the bones, producing early osteoporosis. This new knowledge not only spawned more effective and safer treatments to control RA's inflammation, but also a high priority for prompt and thorough management of the disease. It also focused rheumatologists on preventing atherosclerosis and osteoporosis in RA patients.

It's a miserable fact that less than 50% of atherosclerosis and rheumatoid arthritis patients are currently being treated to these known standards of excellence. It's a miserable fact that we are paying enormous amounts of money to scramble up solu-tions for late complications rather than addressing the risk factors early, dependably, and at a lower cost. Many people cannot get the best care because their insurance won't cover it, or they are not insured at all. Many are underdiagnosed and under-treated because the disease sneaks up slowly and does its dirty work gradually over many years. People who would otherwise be healthy and productive in spite of hav-ing one or more chronic diseases are unable to work and lead a full life. Some recent studies on RA suggest in fact that very early aggressive treatment during a narrow window of opportunity may actually prevent the disease from becoming chronic and destructive at all.

We are paying the high costs of heart failure, joint replacements, care of the dis-abled, lost productivity, and broken relationships rather than controlling chronic diseases early and effectively, and at a lower long-term cost. The victories being achieved for those patients treated as they should be reveal the opportunities being missed for the rest.

It is not only the impact of chronic diseases on our health and economy that draws us to this subject. It is the intriguing and rewarding potential for improving the status quo through redesigning how chronic disease care is provided and paid for. We have much of the required knowledge and technology to diagnose and treat chronic diseases at our fingertips; this is not where the problem lies. The problem is with healthcare delivery and financing. We just haven't put it all together. Redesigning the care of chronic diseases is a commitment that could reenergize those mired in the chaotic US health system, providers, and patients alike, and it is a challenge we cannot afford to neglect. Better health at a lower cost is possible. We are all undernourished from this diet of an oversized bun with little meat – "Where's the beef?"

References

1. Medical Expenditure Panel Survey, 2004. www.ahrq.gov/about/cj2004/meps04.htm. Accessed 24/09/11.
2. CDC.gov/wchs/data/nvsr50/nvsr50_15.pdf. Accessed 24/09/11.
3. Committee on Quality of Health Care in America, Institute of Medicine. Crossing the quality chasm: a new health system for the 21st century. Washington, DC: National Academy Press; 2001.

Chapter 2
How Has the US Health System Evolved?

J. Timothy Harrington

Keywords 20th century healthcare • Scientific medicine • Knowledge • Research • Quality chasm • Chronic disease • Effective care • Training

> *Toto, I've a feeling we're not in Kansas anymore (Dorothy, in the Wizard of Oz).*
> *In 1992, I volunteered to attend a seminar at the Institute of Healthcare Improvement in Boston that introduced me to health system redesign and to Dr. Don Berwick. He asked the 40 or so physicians assembled from across the United States to consider this situation: "You ordered a urinalysis on a patient and came back to the hospital floor later that day to check the result. It wasn't in the chart, so you asked the ward clerk what happened. She said, 'The lab courier picked up the sample this morning. I'll call the lab.'" Back to Dr. Berwick: "What did she tell you the lab said?" The class responded in unison, "They lost the sample." His teaching point was that the problems and errors in any complex system usually happen at the handoffs."*
> J. Timothy Harrington

> *Look at that old photograph.*
> *Is it really you*
> *Smiling like a baby full of dreams?*
> *Smiling ain't so easy now,*
> *Some are coming true.*
> *Nothing's simple as it seems.*
> Kris Kristofferson, This Old Road, C & P 2006, New West
Records, Los Angeles, CA (Fig. 2.1 and Fig. 2.2)

J.T. Harrington, MD (✉)
Division of Rheumatology, University of Wisconsin School of Medicine
and Public Health, Madison, WI, USA
e-mail: timharrington@charter.net

J.T. Harrington and E.D. Newman (eds.), *Great Health Care: Making It Happen*,
DOI 10.1007/978-1-4614-1198-7_2, © Springer Science+Business Media, LLC 2012

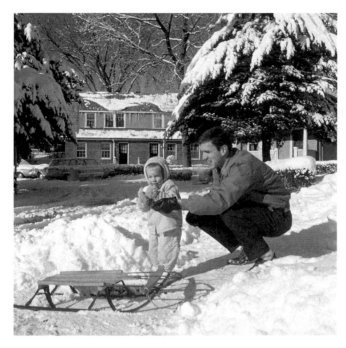

Fig. 2.1 Boston, 1966. Tim Harrington, Medical House Officer with Mark at 18 months

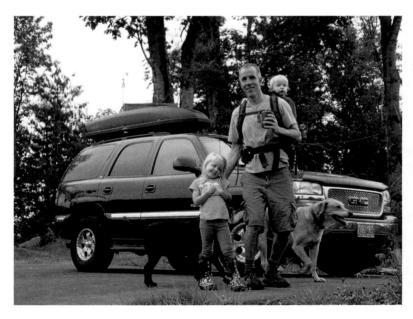

Fig. 2.2 Portland, Oregon, 2010. Mark Harrington, Hospitalist with Ursula, Amelia, Dante, and Mojo

What Was It Like in the "Good Old Days"?

Our understanding of chronic diseases began to change at the dawn of the twentieth century and accelerated in the 1950s. Previously, individual physicians usually provided a diagnosis to explain the patient's symptoms and an estimate of future problems and life expectancy – a prognosis. Diagnostic tests and treatments were limited by today's standards. Patients expected little more from their physicians because this was the way it had always been, and the brighter future of more effective medicine was largely unrecognized. A physician's esteem was derived from his "bedside manner," wisdom, and the acuity of his diagnostic skills. I tell my patients that I have several well-controlled chronic diseases that my grandparents suffered with and died from when they were younger than my present age.

This was the reality when I entered medical school in 1961. Dr. Ben Lawton (Fig. 2.3), a noted Wisconsin surgeon of that era, was fond of saying, "Give me morphine, foxglove (digitalis), and a knife, and I'll do everything for my patient that can be done." The internal medicine specialist of that era worked as an individual with his – rarely her – individual patients, offering diagnosis, prognosis, and comfort. A carefully performed history and physical exam was the tool of the trade that provided clues to the inner workings of the human body, often confirmed or refuted only by postmortem examination. William Osler, the renowned Johns Hopkins

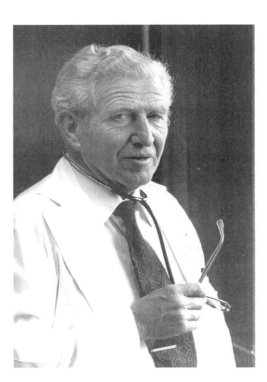

Fig. 2.3 Doctor Ben Lawton (1923–1987). Thoracic surgeon, teacher, founding member of the Marshfield Clinic, Marshfield, WI, and member of the University of Wisconsin Board of Regents

physician, voiced his immortal aphorism in 1898: "Listen to the patient. He's telling you the diagnosis." Medicines and their uses were crude by today's standards. Low potency diuretics, insulin, thyroid pills, and early antibiotics were available, but the stalwart arsenal of today's options did not exist.

Hospitalizations were longer, and in-patient treatments more often than not were limited to nursing care, rest, nutrition, and physical therapy. Patients in heart failure with lungs full of fluid were treated with positive pressure breathing masks and rotating tourniquets to relieve the congestion, we thought. We only had primitive mercurial diuretics to remove their excess fluid. Tubes were placed under the skin in their lower legs to drain edema. Arthritis patients were consigned to weeks of bed rest in hospitals and sanatoria. There, warm water therapy and even hay heated in ovens were applied in a futile attempt to tame the inflammation destroying their joints, and to ease their suffering. Surgery was the answer for many problems that are treated medically today, ulcer disease being one example. The risks of anesthesia and surgery were higher, making this a last resort in many cases. Patients suffered more and died sooner from diseases that can now be held in check or cured – diabetes, rheumatoid arthritis, heart disease, stroke, asthma, and even many cancers.

These were the realities we faced as student doctors then. We could not have imagined the changes we would witness during our professional lifetimes. Many of the "truths" we were taught were based more on our teachers' individual experiences at the bedside and less on formal research. Eminent clinician teachers like William Osler, McGee Harvey, Paul Dudley White, William Middleton, and Walter Bauer became legends. Their seminal clinical observations suggested the basic and clinical research that informs today's medical care. They were the examples of excellence presented to young physicians of my era.

Most 1950s physicians made a living through fee-for-service payments, based on either time spent or procedures performed. Many patients were without insurance and were often cared for with no expectation of payment. When their personal physicians could no longer afford to treat their complex problems, these "charity" patients were referred to public hospitals where physicians-in-training like my contemporaries and me picked up the baton. Measured against today's standards, physicians lived modestly. Many physicians actually resisted Medicare when it came along in the 1960s, though its infusion of new revenues changed physicians' earnings and patients' access to care for the better.

The Emergence of Scientific Medicine

Changes that had been forecast by the isolation of insulin and control of malaria, among others, came more rapidly in the 1950s due to a tipping point in biomedical research. Previous research had emphasized descriptions of clinical symptoms, disease classifications, and studies of human physiology in health and disease. Then biochemistry, molecular biology, and molecular genetics emerged as new scientific disciplines, each contributing profound insights into the causes of diseases and

Table 2.1 Growth of NIH
appropriation 1940–2010

Year	Dollars × 1,000
1940	707
1945	2,835
1950	52,714
1955	81,151
1960	399,380
1965	959,159
1970	1,061,007
1975	2,092,897
1980	3,428,435
1985	5,159,459
1990	7,576,352
1995	11,259,522
2000	17,820,577
2005	28,495,157
2010	31,008,788

Source: National Institutes of Health Office of
Budget. http://officeofbudget.od.nih.gov/approp_
hist.html. Accessed 15/04/11

novel approaches to their treatment. Previous funding of research from private
sources – the Rockefeller and Carnegie Foundations as two examples – was increased
dramatically by commitments from the National Institutes of Health and other fed-
eral agencies. This sustained investment by the American people continues today,
supporting a robust system of medical schools and academic research centers [1]
(Table 2.1).

My first awareness of this research tsunami came during a summer job in 1958
at the University of Wisconsin's McArdle Laboratories under Dr. Charles
Heidelberger. He had synthesized 5FU, a drug that blocked cancer cell growth by
mimicking one of the building blocks of DNA. 5FU became the first effective cancer chemotherapy and is still used today. His home was next door to mine, and he
took an interest in me, becoming a mentor over the earlier years of my medical
career. During one of my medical school assignments several years later, I found
myself giving intravenous 5FU to patients enrolled in cancer research studies. This
was my first personal appreciation of the vital connection between bench research
and bedside patient care.

The explosion of new knowledge gleaned from biomedical research in the last 50
years is beyond comprehension, but a few additional examples will illustrate its
impacts. Unraveling the cholesterol abnormalities that cause atherosclerosis has led
to treatments that delay the onset of heart disease and stroke. Molecular biology
disclosed how cells build their intricate structures, carry out their specialized functions, and communicate with one another. The genetic code was cracked. These
discoveries led in turn to understanding many diseases that are caused by abnormal
functioning of our cells and organs, and how they might be treated.

New chemistry methods enabled scientists to study the body's large molecules
like proteins and fats, whether normal, or altered by abnormal genes or diseases.

Defining the mechanisms of tissue healing and inflammation led to new treatments for arthritis and many other inflammatory diseases, and to preventing rejection of organ transplants. The kidneys' roles in removing waste and balancing fluids and salts were defined, and understanding the failures of these processes in heart and kidney failure led to diuretics, kidney dialysis, and organ transplantation. Vaccines conquered polio and other childhood diseases that were frightening realities for children of my generation and our parents. New antibiotics cured many previously fatal infections. Fiberoptics bent light, allowing physicians to look into the many recesses of the body, and more recently, to perform minimally-invasive surgeries. An expanding array of laboratory and imaging tests produced more precise insights into the functioning and structure of the human body, reducing the emphasis on the physical exam for today's physicians, and on the autopsy for understanding what had gone so wrong for the deceased patient.

The Growing Awareness of the Quality Chasm

These thrilling discoveries and the possibilities they created distracted physicians from the growing evidence in health policy circles during the 1990s that all was not well with health care. In 1996, Vanessa Northington Gamble wrote in the Encyclopedia of the United States in the twentieth century, "A relatively uncomplicated system centered on the individual doctor-patient relationship evolved into a far more intricate one influenced by a myriad of institutions and participants ... factors external to the practice of medicine have profoundly influenced its delivery" [2–4].

In 2001, the Institute of Medicine (IOM) sounded the alarm in a series of reports on the status of health care in the United States, describing an epidemic of avoidable errors, and a "Quality Chasm" that had grown between this profound new scientific knowledge and medical advances on the one hand, and the failure to deliver the best care dependably, efficiently, and safely on the other [5]. The Chasm Report focused on the chronic diseases, their costs, the delays in their diagnosis and treatment, and the frequent errors that often result in irreversible damage to the patient's body and life. The IOM experts defined the problem as a widespread inability of a health system, designed in simpler times, to deliver the best care at the lowest cost in an era of greater complexity. They advocated for fundamental system redesign.

To state it in a slightly different way, the traditional methods, values, and business practices could not cope with the growing options for diagnosis and treatment and technology. Physicians had specialized increasingly to do just that, to cope with it all, but their practices and health systems weren't organized around putting this knowledge to its best uses at the lowest possible costs. Moreover, research has become the highest priority for many medical school faculties – an end unto itself. The goal became to obtain grant funding to create new knowledge, which would in turn support winning more grants. Understanding and improving the delivery of this knowledge lagged behind – a lesser goal. In these environments, physicians-in-training may be steeped in data, but have not learned essential clinical process skills, or how to work in teams.

Table 2.2 United States Healthcare costs, resource use, and outcomes compared to other countries

	Per capita spending ($)	% GNP	Doctors/100,000	Life expectancy
United States	6,719	15.3	26	78
Canada	3,673	10	19	81
Germany	3,465	10.6	34	80
France	3,420	11	23	81
United Kingdom	2,815	8.2	23	80
Italy	2,631	9	37	82
Japan	2,581	8.1	21	83
Russia	698	5.3	43	66
Cuba	674	7.7	59	78
China	216	4.6	14	74

Source: World Health Organization, 2009. www.who.int/whosis/whostat/2009/en/index.htm. Accessed 15/04/11

So we find ourselves in a broken system where …

- Much care is duplicated or unnecessary.
- Insurance companies and many physicians are getting richer while …
- Vital medical care is delayed or omitted.
- The patients and the public are getting sicker and going broke.
- The costs of health care are increasing the national debt beyond redemption.

Our population's health is not what it should be, nor are we doing as well as many other countries, in spite of our far higher costs of care (Table 2.2).

The Distinction Between Being Knowledgeable and Being Effective

From a personal perspective, when I consider the differences between my medical training over 40 years ago and that of younger physicians who have joined my health system in recent years, three differences stand out. First, the dramatic increase in medical school tuition; they have paid 30-fold what I did to get my degree. Second, the imbalance between knowledge and process learning in today's medical schools. And third, the diminished role of experienced clinicians in physicians' training, in particular as related to teaching critical skills for outpatient chronic disease management. As a medical student, I spent considerable time shadowing experienced physicians to observe the nuances of their patient care and the satisfying relationships experienced by physician and patient. This approach is considered less relevant today. Trainees often work with patients alone and then have their work product reviewed by faculty. The same has occurred in nursing education. In my training years, most nurses attended hospital-based programs for 3 years, learning both in the classroom and at the bedside under the tutelage of experienced caregivers. Now they attend 4–5-year degree programs, know much more, but require postgraduate training to develop their hands-on clinical skills.

Table 2.3 Critical questions for clinical quality improvement

Why do it	Benefit for patients
What to do	Research and guidelines
How to do it	Planning, algorithms, PDSA
Who will do it	Defining provider roles and communication
Who will does it work	Tracking key indicators
Who will pay for it	???

We the editors have developed a list of essential questions that should be answered to organize effective health care within local and broader health systems (Table 2.3). Currently, the focus remains disproportionately on what care is best – "What to do?"

Understanding "what to do" is the product of research, and research has been compiled over the last generation into clinical guidelines for managing every chronic disease. So far so good; we have a fat package of necessary information making us smarter. But health care has not improved. That is because we are neglecting the other questions that would make all the difference in helping us to deliver this package to the patient and lead to effectiveness of care, better disease outcomes, and lower cost.

Answering these questions depends on clinical improvement methods more than scientific inquiry. The rest of our book will emphasize these approaches and describe their use.

References

1. Mandel R. Beacon of hope: 1953–1993: The clinical center through 40 years of growth and change in biomedicine. Bethesda, MD: Office of NIH History, National Institutes of Health; 1993.
2. Lederer SE. Medical science and technology. In: Kutler SI, editor. Encyclopedia of the United States in the twentieth century, vol. 2. New York, NY: Charles Scribner's Sons; 1996. p. 941–56.
3. Meckel RA. Health and disease. In: Kutler SI, editor. Encyclopedia of the United States in the twentieth century, vol. 2. New York, NY: Charles Scribner's Sons; 1996. p. 957–86.
4. Gamble VN. Health care delivery. In: Kutler SI, editor. Encyclopedia of the United States in the twentieth century, vol. 2. New York, NY: Charles Scribner's Sons; 1996. p. 987–1007.
5. Committee on Quality of Health Care in America, Institute of Medicine. Crossing the quality chasm: a new health system for the 21st century Washington. Washington, DC: National Academy Press; 2001.

Chapter 3
Why Has the US Health System Become What It Is?

J. Timothy Harrington

Keywords U.S. Health system • Ineffective • Health care providers • Variation • Cookbook medicine • Fee-for-service payment • Fragmented care • Zero sum game

> We can't solve problems by using the same kind of thinking we used when we created them
>
> Albert Einstein.

> In 1960, I landed a summer job at the Oscar Mayer factory in Madison, working on a production line with five full-time employees. Our job was to package hot dogs, 12 to a pack. We were paid a base salary depending on years of service and a bonus not to exceed 15% if we churned out 15% more packages than the standard. If we did still better, the bosses would re-set the standard, and the bonus would decrease – same salary, less bonus, more work. Regular as clockwork, our line generated between 113–117% of standard, day after day. I figured out pretty quickly that the other workers could have produced twice as much product, with or without me, but the company got the volume it needed and the employees got the extra pay they needed for doing as much work as was necessary, no less and no more.

> Paying physicians fee-for-service seems at first like the way I got paid for packing hot dogs, but it's different in important ways. There is no ceiling on how much I can earn. The incentive is to pack in the greatest volume of health care I can manage of services that pay the most per unit. And there is no incentive for teamwork (I still can't stomach hot dogs, but that's another story).
>
> J. Timothy Harrington.

J.T. Harrington, MD (✉)
Division of Rheumatology, University of Wisconsin School of Medicine
and Public Health, Madison, WI, USA
e-mail: timharrington@charter.net

J.T. Harrington and E.D. Newman (eds.), *Great Health Care: Making It Happen*,
DOI 10.1007/978-1-4614-1198-7_3, © Springer Science+Business Media, LLC 2012

Why has the US Health System become what it is? Why have we failed to respond to the explosion of knowledge and technology by inventing or adopting processes aimed at more reliable delivery? In Dr. Don Berwick's words, the handoffs have multiplied and we aren't managing them effectively – more options, more physicians and other providers involved, and long years of treatment during which events and decisions pile one upon the other.

In our opinion, there are several root causes.

* Health care provider perspectives
* Fee-for-service payments for fragments of care
* The zero sum game of health care economics

Healthcare Provider Perspectives

The dominant values of people working inside the system – physicians, hospital administrators, and others – emphasize independence, individualism, competition, and profits. These values are deeply rooted in US healthcare, as they are in our society more generally. This is the American Way, where relatively little attention is paid to teamwork or a sense of the common good. Our health care is uniquely expensive and ineffective compared to other developed (and even not so developed) countries where they manage medical care as a public resource, like roads, and police, and fire departments.

Despite evidence to the contrary, many physicians will tell you that traditional "mom and pop" practices are still capable of shepherding their patients through today's healthcare labyrinth. We learned this model in medical school, many of us still believe it, and it is not so. We were also taught that we bear sole responsibility for the outcomes of care; that bad outcomes equal bad physicians, rather than good people working in bad systems.

Individualism – doing it my way – leads to high process variation that precludes excellent and efficient delivery of services. This is true in any business, though most physicians look at their profession as unique. They adhere to the methods they learned in their medical training and resist process standardization as "cookbook medicine." If the recipe is flawed, then I agree that cookbook medicine is unsavory. But if the recipe uses high quality ingredients and has been tested, then it is worth retaining and repeating – indeed, our well-being depends on it.

Most of what patients need to have done can in fact be standardized. Exceptions should only be recognized in this context. The handoffs become chaotic when providers are playing by different sets of rules. Errors and costs multiply in such environments. What patient has not been given conflicting opinions and instructions from multiple physicians within the same health system or specialty? As another example, hospitals in my community maintained inventories of several different brands of total joint replacement hardware based on each orthopedic surgeon's personal preference. The avoidable excess cost of this lack of standardization exceeded a million dollars per year, per hospital.

Insurers and their allied benefit management companies have recently challenged the roles of physicians as the "deciders" in order to themselves influence what care is delivered, how, and by whom. We are buried in paperwork: precertification of services, denials of payments for "unnecessary" or purportedly "investigational" care, and medicine formularies. And the demands change per insurer. My office, for example, wrestles daily with fifteen different insurer sets of regulations and forms. We get no extra pay or pats on the back for what is truly excessive time- and effort-involved.

From the viewpoint of an individual insurance company, these rules and regulations appear structured to cut short-term (not long-term) costs, to streamline their internal work product, and to maximize their revenue. To those of us working directly with patients, however, it's a white-out blizzard with little redemptive value. Certainly variation in patient populations is not respected. The present insurance system, in fact, contributes to a very real "cookbook medicine" world that undermines sound professional judgment and best patient care. Good doctors all over this country worry about this, talk about it, and fight it however and whenever they can.

Some of these burdens can be viewed as a response to the failure of physicians to adopt more efficient, effective processes ourselves. I don't dispute that. But what's also indisputable is the end result: an increased workload for providers and no documented improvement in overall healthcare delivery or costs.

Payment for Fragments of Care

A second cause of the problems that permeate the US health system is fee-for-service payment to healthcare providers – payment to individual providers for fragments of care. The origins of fee-for-service go back to the 1930s, before health insurance existed. Individual physicians and surgeons provided all the care that was available for most conditions and billed the patients directly – a simple methodology for a much simpler environment.

Today, fee-for-service is an artifact; or it should be. The healthcare environment has changed dramatically around this now antiquated process. It still rewards the volume of services, but with no relation to clinical outcomes or efficiency. Procedures in general, and select other services, enjoy high compensation relative to those related to overseeing long-term care for chronic diseases. By paying for fragments of service, fee-for-service offers no incentives for teamwork, for completing sequences of services required to produce desired outcomes, and for physicians and patients to take the long view.

As one example, the goal of osteoporosis care is to prevent fractures related to bone fragility that occur with aging and certain diseases. In people over 50, one fracture increases the risk of future fractures, so they enter into a long-term compact with their fracture risk. We now have the capabilities to identify those at high risk, treat them effectively, and ensure the vital continuum of this treatment for many years.

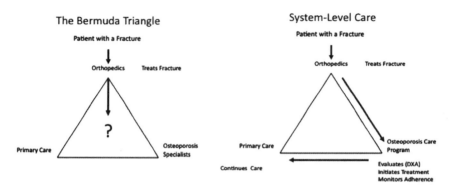

Fig. 3.1 Redesigning osteoporosis care to achieve reliability and reduced fracture

Fee-for-service is not our friend in this relationship. It wastes money paying certain specialists who aren't adequately trained to diagnose or treat osteoporosis; it fails to reward good outcomes; it doesn't support long-term follow-up. And so, too many osteoporotic patients are not getting the best care. Many studies agree that treating fractures is more expensive than preventing them and that Medicare – read, the American taxpayer – bears much of the cost of this undermanagement.

This typically fragmented approach to osteoporosis can be characterized as a Bermuda Triangle (Fig. 3.1) in which the orthopedic surgeon treats the patient's fracture – what he or she gets paid to do – and then the patient "disappears" forever. We heartily concur with health policy experts who suggest this will only change when fee-for-service payment is abandoned in favor of paying accountable care organizations (ACOs) globally for the entire episode of care and better outcomes. In Chap. 14, Dr. Richard Dell will describe just such a coordinated and reliable ACO system and how it reduced fractures in people with osteoporosis.

Fee-for-service has influenced the US health system because it rewards physicians and hospitals for doing more of what produces the highest revenues. Physicians and hospitals, like all humans, respond to how we are paid. Fee-for-service pressures become even greater in smaller medical practices where the physician's income is the net of revenues less expenses. In a physician group that I was part of once, this was called "turning the crank."

Another poorly recognized consequence of fee-for-service payment relates to the difference between hands-on and downstream revenues. The former are performed directly by the provider for the patient; the latter are ordered by the provider but performed by others, like X-rays and lab tests. Downstream revenue varies dramatically from as little as 10% for many surgeons to as much as 50% for internal medicine specialists who provide chronic disease management. If downstream revenues are paid to the physician who orders the services in the first place, as in small practices with their own labs and X-ray machines, they order more of them. A prominent rheumatologist in an independent practice said not long ago that, "I pay my office expenses with my patient care revenues, and take home the profits from my laboratory and x-ray business." At the other extreme, if physician compensation is based

Table 3.1 Public and private medical school tuition and trainee debt

Year	Annual tuition (median $)		Graduate debt (median $)	
	Public	Private	Public	Private
1984	5,231	20,939	22,000	27,000
2003	16,322	34,550	100,000	135,000

Source: Jolly P. Medical school tuition and young physicians' indebtedness. Health Affairs 2005;24:527–535

only on hands-on payments, as is true in many larger medical groups, internal medical specialists are disadvantaged relative to procedural physicians. This helps to explain why so many internists practice in single-specialty groups that have their own office labs and imaging facilities. The trade-off is a vital one: higher income for the single-specialty group; less integrated care management of the patients.

The spiral of unintended consequences from fee-for-service payment goes on and on. The "more is better" rationale has been adopted by many providers and sold to patients, in spite of the documented risks and costs of excessive intervention in many cases. We have more MRI's and spine surgery because these are big money-makers for the hospitals and physicians themselves, and once in place, these resources are bound to be used to the limit. In contrast, less expensive self-care, preventive, and rehabilitative approaches are underutilized. The business model of fixed resource costs and volume-based revenues drive the utilization of these expensive diagnostic technologies and procedures.

The current generations of medical graduates who are burdened with higher educational debt than their predecessors understand these economics very well. In the 1950s and 1960s, many physicians chose the excitement of scientifically based internal medicine. Not so today. Procedural capabilities and profits have escalated along with medical tuitions (Table 3.1), causing shifts to the higher-paid surgical and medical procedural specialties. We are left with an imbalance in physician manpower that cannot be corrected in the short run or in the current physician compensation environment.

In this analysis, the insurance industry is not to blame for fee-for-service because this is how most physicians have been paid going way back. Many physicians have supported its continuation, especially those who are the winners. The HMO movement of the 1980s was undermined by the fee-for-service mentality. Even though medical groups and independent physician associations (IPAs) received a global payment for each patient's care, the monies were too often distributed internally among providers based on traditional fee-for-service, piecework schemes. This disconnect led physicians to compete with one another for a larger share of the pie by doing more of whatever they did, and the insurance companies were forced to pass on premium increases driven by physician expectations to the businesses that purchased the care for employees and their families. The expected teamwork and efficiencies in delivery of care did not materialize because the incentives of capitated payments were undermined by physicians' adherence to fee-for-service competitive thinking.

The Zero Sum Game

Finally, we must recognize that very powerful stakeholders have shaped the US health system to their own advantage. The 2009–2010 health reform debate was driven by these players, and their behaviors of self-interest and entitlement were well characterized as a "zero sum game" in "Redefining Health Care," a 2006 book by Michael Porter and Elizabeth Teisberg, two well-known US economists [1].

The zero sum game has each healthcare stakeholder competing against the others for their own greater success, but with little interest in cooperating, and with little respect for the interests of patients and our society. This is a uniquely American approach to health care, as we have mentioned already; so is our tolerance of health care as a business and an opportunity for profit. Other countries are doing better with less because their stakeholder interests are better aligned and their sense of the common good is stronger. It is easier for them to expand funding and capacity within their better-organized systems than it is for us to improve our underperforming and already overfunded health system. And how ironic that we view biomedical research as an essential public investment, but not the delivery of its discoveries to the benefit of the citizens who have financed it! Porter and Teisberg do not suggest, however, that competition should be removed from the US health system, but instead that the stakeholders should be rewarded for improving the value of care, defined as better long-term outcomes at a lower cost.

Dr. Atul Gawande writing in The New Yorker exposed the high variance in Medicare costs across different communities in the United States that has everything to do with personal gain and bad habits, and nothing to do with patient benefit [2]. Dr. Elliot Fisher's research at Dartmouth Medical School indicated that McAllen, Texas is the most expensive city for Medicare patients in the US, far more costly than El Paso right up the road. These authors suggest that McAllen physicians have designed their practices as profit centers for maximizing revenues that then support their other entrepreneurial medical and independent business interests. In other areas, physicians are just in the habit of ordering a lot more of the care that provides no benefit, and in fact, patients generally do worse in these communities.

An Institute of Medicine white paper, "Reducing Costs through the Appropriate Use of Specialty Services" documents a $700 billion burden of overuse in US health care, 30% of total direct costs [3]. Overuse is defined as "clinical care that appears to be excessively utilized given the known tradeoffs between its costs plus potential harms compared to its potential benefits." Overuse and excessive costs vary by community and relate most frequently to the lack of evidence supporting a service. Where evidence is relatively weak, high variance and overuse are common. In contrast, where evidence is strong, underutilization is the more commonly observed deviation from optimal care. These well-documented observations suggest that high value care will depend on a combination of realizing savings from higher efficiency and a decrease in overuse, and then reallocating these savings to providing necessary but underutilized services (Fig. 3.2).

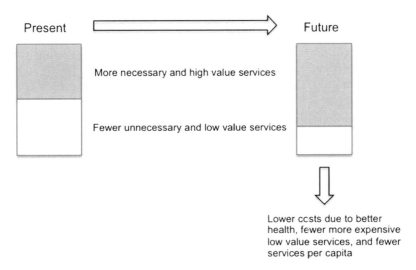

Fig. 3.2 Improving the value and cost of health care

Consider the ads in daily newspapers and on TV that are all about encouraging people to seek out expensive elective services. Both for-profit and not-for-profit hospital systems compete for market share, using new technologies and vying for the loyalty of "rainmaker" physicians. The costs of duplicative facilities and technologies not only include initial acquisition and construction, but also the inevitable increased utilization of these new beds, ORs, and machines.

Government efforts to consolidate facilities, technologies, and services are often undermined by competing stakeholders. Efforts to inject public interest into this competition through "certificate of need" laws haven't worked, though a few notable exceptions exist. Where healthcare communities cooperate to reduce waste – such as in Richmond, Virginia and Grand Junction, Colorado – costs have decreased more than a little. In addition, hospitals that provide higher volumes of services for specific diseases are known to achieve better outcomes and lower costs of care. So why do low volume hospitals continue to do business in the same communities?

Where Does This Leave Physicians and Our Patients?

Individualism, fee-for-service incentives that encourage high volumes of care and favor more profitable services, and the "zero sum game" are all extracting a price from doctors and patients. At a time when cooperation to improve delivery of care is needed, many physicians are running harder and harder to maintain their incomes. This has been aptly characterized as "hamster health care" by Ian Morrison and Richard Smith in their 2002 *British Medical Journal* editorial: more patients, more services, less time available, and higher administrative burdens. Many physicians see no way to influence the forces that are shaping their practices, or how they can afford to change for the better. The majority supported healthcare reform, but are troubled about how to manage the time, work, and resources required to maintain – much less reform – the way they practice medicine.

Physicians are not all squeaky clean either. We are attuned to our financial performance, but do not regularly measure the disease status of patients and the outcomes or costs of care. Even when we do, we do not reliably address these problems. This "medical inertia" has been studied thoroughly by Dr. Lawrence Phillips, and it is clear that physicians do not treat uncontrolled chronic conditions like high blood pressure and diabetes as aggressively as needed [4]. The impact of this undermanagement is profound. Once again, the patient suffers and the long-term costs skyrocket.

Unless we fundamentally redesign how care is delivered and how we are paid, change will be incremental at best. It is no accident that the emerging examples of great health care, including those provided in our book, have been developed more frequently in integrated systems where resources and provider compensation are focused on teamwork, coordination of services, efficiency, better patient outcomes and satisfaction, and yes, profitability.

References

1. Porter ME, Teisberg EO. Redefining health care: creating value-based compensation on results. Boston, MA: Harvard Business School Press; 2006.
2. Gawande A. The cost conundrum, The New Yorker, June 1, 2009.
3. Baker N, Whittington JW, Resar RK, Griffin FA, Nolan KM. Reducing costs through the appropriate use of specialty services. IHI Innovation Series white paper, Institute for Healthcare Improvement. Cambridge, MA: 2010. www.IHI.org.
4. Phillips LS, Twombly JG. It's time to overcome clinical inertia. Ann Intern Med. 2008; 148:783–5.

Chapter 4
Making Chronic Disease Care Great

J. Timothy Harrington

Keywords Great health care • Change • Alignment • Team care • Care coordination

> When you're in a hole, stop digging (*Denis Healey, a British Labor politician, presented this "first law of holes".) (Fig. 4.1). When Felix Frankfurter was an eminent professor of law at Harvard in the 1920's, one of his students, Adolph Berle, attended Frankfurter's course two years in a row. "What, back again?" Frankfurter asked. "I wanted to see if you'd learned anything," Berle replied*
> (*Source: Amity Shlaes. The Forgotten Man: a new history of the great depression.*).
> *Our goal must be to identify the combination of essential delivery system 'production' factors that can consistently deliver care of greatest value for patients over the lifetime of their illnesses*
> (*David M. Lawrence, MD, CEO, Kaiser Permanente, Annals of Internal Medicine, 2005.*).

Lots of Proposals, No Simple Answers

The authors of this book believe that advocating for the status quo is unacceptable. The assertion that we have "the best health system in the world" ignores copious statistical evidence to the contrary, as well as the less quantifiable but critically relevant stress and suffering of physicians and patients caught in the current chaos. Our challenge: getting from where we are to a better future by skillfully managing change.

J.T. Harrington, MD (✉)
Division of Rheumatology, University of Wisconsin School of Medicine
and Public Health, Madison, WI, USA
e-mail: timharrington@charter.net

J.T. Harrington and E.D. Newman (eds.), *Great Health Care: Making It Happen*,
DOI 10.1007/978-1-4614-1198-7_4, © Springer Science+Business Media, LLC 2012

Fig. 4.1 Troutdale, Oregon, 2009. Doctors Mark and Tim Harrington filling in holes

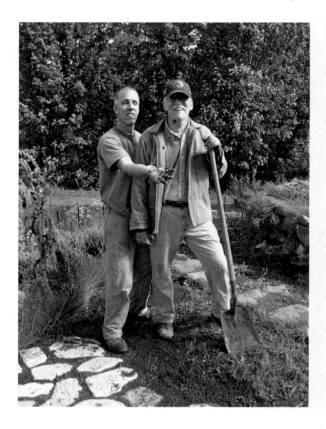

Dr. Atul Gawande provided a compelling analogy recently in his New Yorker article *Testing, Testing*. "To figure out how to transform medical communities, with all their diversity and complexity, is going to involve trial and error. And this will require pilot programs – lots of them" [1].

From Dr. Gawande's perspective, the many proposals being advocated for improving healthcare outcomes and costs should be viewed as testable opportunities, and only attempted if they are focused on informing significant improvement rather than protecting self-interests. In the 2010 health reform legislation, money has been allocated for three quality improvement functions Dr. Gawande identifies as pivotal to great health care: process testing; comparative effectiveness research; and expert advisory committees to guide physicians and patients toward higher value decisions.

Immediate improvements are reasonable to expect from process testing. Medicare's 5-year "meaningful use" initiative stakes out guideposts [2]. It encourages practices to adopt electronic medical records and to use them for electronic prescribing, communication with other providers, and improving care. Practices will also be asked to measure and report specific outcomes of care for their Medicare patients. Government financial incentives will support and encourage these improvements, just as government support for research kindled the bonfire of new medical knowledge in the twentieth century.

In contrast, expecting we can improve health care by pumping up medical school enrollment seems to us a flawed prospect. We certainly cannot address the baby-boomer demographic by simply growing the physician work force. It will cost more, take years to have an impact, and offer no guarantees. Chapter 2, Table 2.2 documented the weak relationships across countries between the numbers of physicians per capita and both the costs of health care and life expectancies. No number of physicians doing what we are doing now will make things better. Future physicians must be given the tools to manage continuous, positive change, and once armed with that knowledge, they'll need to find places to use it. That means health systems that are already engaged in continuous, positive change. More on this in Chap. 26.

Better to begin redesigning care first and make an informed decision at a later date on the optimal number of physicians, nurses, and other providers. Otherwise, we're just guessing at a solution to a problem we don't yet understand. Process testing will not only be required to determine how care can be best delivered, but also how the workforce should be organized to do it: the how and the who of improving systems (Chap. 2, Fig. 2.1). For example, younger physicians are more commonly working fewer hours, and often part-time. Emergency rooms and urgent care centers are inadequate stopgaps – we ve been there and tried that. More effective alternatives need to be tested, such as job-sharing by teams of part-time physicians to collectively provide full days and weeks of access to primary care. This is how many specialty practices function already, and where this has been tried in primary care, patients love it. And how many primary physicians will be needed as hospitalists assume their inpatient responsibilities and midlevel providers are fully utilized.

Patients want great health care. So do most of us who work in today's broken-down health system. It's just that we're mired in the mud of it. This happens in any failing organization, as Robert Quinn described in his 1996 business book, "Deep Change". Borrowing Quinn's perspective, physicians face three choices: to relocate or quit, to stay put and fail along with their organizations, or to stand up and work for positive change. A different practice location or a move to industry or administration too often turns out to be more of the same because the current problems are pervasive, while retirement deprives the physician of the rewards of serving patients, and the patients of their physicians. So we go along to get along. There's no happy ending in this response either; it only prolongs the suffering. Quinn suggests that only the third alternative – standing up and working for positive change – is both rational and rewarding for physicians, our local health systems, our patients, and society. We currently have too few physicians choosing option three.

Our Vision

It's simple. The editors and authors of this book have chosen to stand up and work for positive change. We believe the road maps to a brighter future are to be found in those examples of great care that have generally developed in environments where the game is not "zero sum," where interests of insurers, providers, and patients are better aligned, where team care is the standard, value is defined by the better health in patient populations, and lower costs are a priority. The stakeholders in these practices and health systems live by the Cleveland Clinic's mantra of putting "Patients First."

In Part II, Dr. Newman will provide the tools for today's physicians to begin performing this important work, and tomorrow's to hit the ground running. In Part III, we will review various aspects of improving chronic disease care. In Part IV," our champions will describe how they provide great health care for different chronic diseases, what motivated them, and how they built and are sustaining their programs. Finally, in Part V, we will discuss controversies that are obstructing change, and how these might be resolved positively. Read on.

References

1. Gawande A. Testing, testing. The New Yorker, January 2010.
2. www.cms.govEHRincentiveprograms. Accessed 2 April 2011.

Part II
How to Effect Change in Health Care: If It Doesn't Fit, Use a Larger Hammer

Eric D. Newman

I am reminded of one of my favorite movies, "Young Frankenstein" (Mel Brooks, 1974). The subject matter is nothing short of the creation of life from inanimate protoplasm. There is a poignant scene, where Professor Frankenstein (pronounced 'frahn-ken-steen"), the grandson of the original Dr. Frankenstein, is seeking his grandfather's secret laboratory where he created the first "monster". After searching through secret doors and passageways, he happens upon the laboratory, and there on the table is his grandfather's diary, containing the secret of the creation of life. The camera pans to the diary's cover, which simply reads, "How I did it".

This part is devoted to the techniques needed to completely redesign the delivery of health care for patients with chronic disease. That's all. A relatively simple task to be sure. We promise that after reading this section, it will be crystal clear how to do it – how to create great health care. Or my name isn't Frahnkensteen.

E.D. Newman, MD
Department of Rheumatology,
Clinical Innovations.
Division of Medicine,
Geisinger Health System,
Danville, PA, USA

Chapter 5
Building Systems of Care

Eric D. Newman

Keywords Systems of care • Chronic disease • System dynamics • Clinical micro-system • Non-adoptors • Improvement • System • System behavior • Change a system

"It was hot outside so my dog ate my BMW."
Yes, this is a true story. More importantly, it symbolizes one of the most important concepts surrounding systems, and why we commonly fail to effectively effect change. Within a system, a set of very logical changes often leads to an illogical end result. Read on.
We recently adopted a 9-month-old yellow Labrador retriever named Cooper. Cooper quickly learned the boundaries of his invisible fence, which ends halfway across our driveway. As with most labs, Cooper likes to scavenge within his territory. If it moves, smells, or essentially has the physical properties of a liquid, solid, (or sometimes gas), its fair game for licking, chewing, (or inhaling).
It was unusually hot outside 3 weeks ago, so my wife Laurie moved our van from the driveway into my usual space in the garage. My daughter's boyfriend Justin arrived and parked in the driveway behind the van. I drove home and parked next to Justin in the driveway (now within Cooper's invisible fence territory) because hey, it was either that or the grass.

E.D. Newman, MD (✉)
Department of Rheumatology, Clinical Innovations, Division of Medicine,
Geisinger Health System, Danville, PA, USA
e-mail: arthman@aol.com

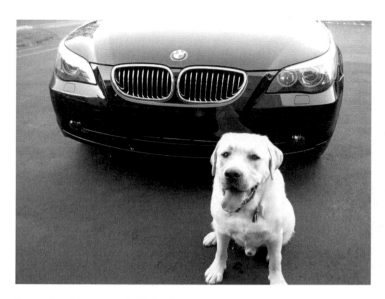

Fig. 5.1 Cooper inquiring as to what's for dessert

Later that evening, Cooper (who was inside most of the day because of the heat) started bugging the heck out of Laurie. An animal lover who finally lost her cool, Laurie escorted Cooper outside and asked him to go play nicely by himself for a while (a rough translation of the actual exchange). Twenty minutes later, Laurie looked out the window, and with a horrified look on her face, uttered the phrase no self-respecting man ever wants to hear .... "Cooper, stop eating the BMW!!!" (Fig. 5.1). A set of logical changes led to an illogical conclusion. And a hefty repair bill, as well as orthodontics.

For this chapter, I will orient the reader to systems, how they fit in the context of health care, and illustrate the respect one must have for perturbing a system, lest one winds up enduring a similar fate as my poor car.

Eric D. Newman

Patients with chronic disease require care that is highly dependable and accessible. They need to be monitored for disease activity and have their disease controlled by treatments that strike the best balance between efficacy and safety. They need this to occur now (actual yesterday) – not wait 15 years until we can transform best knowledge into routine best practice.

So what's the problem? For starters, the physicians and coproviders of care for patients with chronic diseases are challenged by the additional requirements for preventive care and acute care, the need for management of coexisting conditions that cross specialties and expanse of time, and a mass of information that is expanding at a rate beyond our abilities to easily manage. For finishers, there simply aren't enough of us around to effectively and efficiently manage all of a patient's needs in the healthcare model we have today – everything gets done at a face-to-face visit, or it doesn't get done. Precisely!

So what do we want? Health care that is safe, timely, effective, efficient, equitable, and patient-centric [1]. To achieve this goal for large numbers of patients, there needs to be a fundamental redesign of how we provide care. It starts with an understanding, and respect, for systems.

What's a System and Does It Bite?

A system is defined as a set of elements (pieces ... parts) that work together to achieve a common goal [2]. These parts are interdependent – they interact with one another. To make it more interesting, each "part" may itself be a system. A system within a system within a system – kind of like those wooden Russian Babushka nesting dolls. In health care, we are talking about systems that involve sentient beings, commonly referred to as humans. Highly complex, unpredictable, strong-willed, moody, and irrational on a good day, they are the perfect ingredient to make systems even more complicated and unpredictable.

Systems can by their nature contain properties not found in their individual parts. For example, letters by themselves may be meaningless, but when placed together can form something with new meaning – a word. Words can form sentences (new meaning beyond the individual words). Sentences can form stanzas, stanzas can form Sonnets, and pretty soon everyone is making love. And that's how babies are born.

If we want to understand how systems behave, we can turn to the science of System Dynamics – where understanding the structure of a system may help us understand the behavior of that system. If we want to play in systems and redesign them, we need to consider Systems Thinking. This way of viewing the world includes three concepts:

1. A belief that the parts of a system behave differently by themselves than they do as part of the system
2. By teasing apart how the parts interact with one another, we can better understand a system
3. Many systems are complex – crossing space and time – so a small change at one end can lead to large and unpredictable consequences at the other end. Think about the "whisper game," where you have a group of people in a line. The first person whispers a phrase into the ear of the second person in line, then that person whispers what they thought they heard to the third person, and so on. There is always some wise guy in the middle who deliberately changes the phrase in ways no one could predict. At the end of the game, the last person tells what they heard, and the first person tells what they said. Such a game might start with the phrase "A horse is a horse of course of course", and end with the proclamation

"When the chips are down, the buffalo is empty." Systems are complex, and perturbing them leads to unexpected outcomes.

In health care, and in every day life, we tend to think in very traditional terms – that events occur in a very linear fashion. "A" causes "B" which results in "C." I order a test. The test is then performed and resulted. The results are placed in my patient's chart. Systems thinking requires us to consider complex interactive terms. Information and action flow in two directions. Parts interact with one another along the way. We have inputs, outputs, processes, feedback, and controls to consider. I order a test. The patient takes the test order to the front desk. The patient may tell the front desk they want to go the lab today here, or they want to go today somewhere else, to go in the future when they want to, to coordinate my request with other blood drawing that may or may not yet be rescheduled, or maybe they refuse because it's too costly. Information is fed back to me later that day that the patient left already, refused the lab work, and what do I want to do? Whew – I didn't even get past "the test was ordered!"

Healthcare Systems, Systems-Based Care and Bears (oh my)

So what's a system in health care? A system may be the process of treating someone with diabetes. Or testing a new treatment for hypertension. A system could also be a Rheumatology Clinic. The good folks at Dartmouth would call this a clinical microsystem. A clinical microsystem is a small group of people, who together work to provide healthcare to a group of patients. The characteristics of a clinical microsystem are that it has certain goals from a business and clinical perspective, information is shared within the system, the microsystem produces certain outcomes, the microsystem can change over time, and it is usually part of some larger health system.

At first glance, this would seem intuitive. Yet we as healthcare providers do not typically consider ourselves to be part of a system. We call ourselves nurses, doctors, secretaries, front desk staff, and administrators. Doctors do doctor stuff, secretaries do secretary stuff, administrators do (fill in the blank). We do not identify ourselves based in the system we function, nor do we consider ourselves as part of a smaller system within a large system designed to deliver (poor to fair) medical care. When you ask a physician specialist, "what do you do?," you get the response "I specialize in diseases of the rich" (to quote Tom Lehrer). You don't hear "I am part of a highly organized health care team that is designed to provide the best care possible at the greatest value for those we serve – our patients." What a different world it would be if we thought in those terms and acted accordingly.

A systems-based care approach is not an option, it's a necessity, if we are going to provide care that exudes quality and respects cost and resource utilization.

System Core Principles and Characteristics

"Every System is perfectly designed to achieve the results it achieves" [3]. The system of health care we have designed, where we reward doing more rather than doing better, is perfectly designed to ratchet the cost up exponentially with little regard to the consequences (since in most instances we don't objectively monitor the results). Not quite sure I understand why people are continually surprised at this. Probably not system thinkers! Fortunately, you as the reader are far more enlightened. Read on McDuff.

Huber [4] helps us pull our understanding of systems together succinctly by outlining some core principles:

1. Every system needs a purpose. It may be nefarious and evil, or saintly and beneficent, or just practical.
2. A system's performance is determined by its structure. Ever wonder why only 10% of your patients arrive with the information you need to provide best care? Try examining the structure of your system for scheduling new patient visits. The answer is in the flow.
3. Bad things can happen when you change a system's structure. Let's call that a Cooperism.
4. Structure also determines who benefits. Important to consider as successful system redesign will leave some constituencies doing better, and others worse off.
5. Degree of improvement is a function of a system's size and scope. Big system – big gains possible. Or big problems.
6. Systems require cooperation. It should be obvious (but isn't) that since the pieces and parts of systems are interdependent, that cooperation between these parts is crucial.
7. Systems need to be managed. Simply changing a system will not result in sustained improvement. Systems need to be groomed, fed, watered, and walked periodically.
8. Leadership within systems is paramount. While there are well-described spontaneous events (like human combustion – go ahead, Google it), systems don't spontaneously improve themselves. Improvement changes within a system need to lead, or the system will continue down its merry path of either continued poor performance, or massive self-destruction. But put a "Change Champion" at the helm, someone trusted and respected by the System's players (parts), someone that can define the issues, set the expectations, and facilitate the process, and great things can be done.

If we understand and believe these core principles, then what constitutes a "really well-oiled system"? Huber also describes the following characteristics as being associated with high-performing Clinical Microsystems:

1. Leadership that is strong
2. Support within the organization
3. Focus on staff, training, performance, process improvement

4. Focus on the patient, the community, and the market
5. Care teams that rely on each other
6. Effective use of information and information technology

So here's the quick summary – systems need a purpose and a leader, they need to be managed and respected, and understanding the system's structure is paramount.

How to Change a System: The Wrong Way and the Right Way

How many of us have been part of a well-meaning steering committee, where on a cold January morning we discussed with great emotion the vicissitudes of life, and conclude that we earnestly need to immediately operationalize across our system the requirement that all physicians begin night clinics – only to find out 6 months later that we have lost hundreds of thousands of dollars in added staffing expense, because few patients showed up. Committees in general are not set up to redesign systems effectively. Take the dead horse analogy, for example.

The tribal wisdom of the Dakota Indians, passed on from generation to generation, says that, "When you discover that you are riding a dead horse, the best strategy is to dismount." This is a wise and prudent thing to do.

In healthcare, more advanced strategies are often employed, such as

- Buying a stronger whip
- Changing riders
- Appointing a committee to study the horse
- Arranging visits to see how others ride horses
- Lowering the standards so that dead horses can be included
- Promoting the dead horse to a supervisory position
- Hiring outside contractors to ride the dead horse
- Doing a productivity study to see if lighter riders would improve the dead horse's performance
- Declaring that as the dead horse does not have to be fed, it is less costly, carries lower overhead, and therefore contributes substantially more to the bottom line than do some other horses (and my favorite)
- Reclassifying the dead horse as living-impaired

And while you may laugh (and we hope you do), a certain part of this rings true, doesn't it? We change systems without considering that we are in a system. We solve problems by getting people in a room and gaining consensus. Changing a system for the better requires effective problem-solving skills – more on this in Chap. 6.

Remember Dr. Berwick's quote "Every System is perfectly designed to achieve the results it achieves." With that in mind, we need to consider what result we want to achieve, then be thoughtful about the process we utilize. But because we often solve problems while simultaneously ignoring the system-ness of health care, we tend to create workarounds rather than truly redesigning and improving the system of care.

As an example let's take the problem that many new patients we see are missing important information. The result is we get delayed trying to track the information down, or perhaps unnecessary tests are performed. So our solution of course is to simply put down an edict – if the patient arrives without x, y, and z, we will not see them. Indeed, in some sense, you did solve the problem – now virtually 100% of the patient you see have the needed info (they were of course the ones that would have come with the info anyway). The unintended consequence is that you did not bother to understand the process that results in patient's not arriving with the information, and essentially have now refused to see 50% of your referrals. The patients are unhappy, the referring docs are shouting your name and burning you in effigy, and you are forced to retire earlier than expected.

What would be a better way? Begin by understanding the system of obtaining information about new patients. Flow it out, and you would find a tangled gnarly mess of miscommunication, dropped balls, variability, and general brouhaha. A process ripe for simplification and redesign!

The Challenge

I can sum this up in 1 word – "people." It is often said that an administrator's job would be much easier if it weren't for the people. Of course I have also heard the reverse. I can teach the skill set of learning how to effectively effect change, redesign, and create large successful programs that are effective and efficient. But I can't change behavior, at least not easily.

And while I am blessed to live in an environment and work in a department with a few innovators and many who are willing to change if the case is made, I have also encountered my fair share of nonadoptors. How do you spot a nonadoptor? It's easy. Just listen for the following quotes:

We're too busy
Everyone else is backlogged
My waiting list means that I am that good
We've been doing it this way for years
This is just about administration trying to get me to see more patients
You're just rearranging the deck chairs on the Titanic …

My suggestions for how to deal with nonadoptors? Ignore them, fire them, or if they are your boss, go work somewhere else. Because a sea of change is coming. The process improvement freaks will inherit the earth. And to quote the Borg, "Resistance is futile."

Lessons Learned

I would like to finish with some concepts Dr. Berwick brings to light in his primer on leading improvements in systems.

- You cannot create sustainable improvement by fiat. Simply saying it will be so will not make it happen. You want to improve by changing the system rather than changing within the system. As an example, we cannot ultimately improve care by simply seeing more patients and doing more to them – that is changing within the (failed) system.
- Have specific aims in mind and don't try to have too many balls in the air. Would you rather do 20 things poorly or two things really well?
- If you want to gain understanding, you need to measure. And don't aim for a perfect measure, or to develop a perfect system. Really good is a good start.
- Find great ideas. And keep in mind, they may come from sources you may previously have not engaged – what about your costaff (nurses, front desk, staff, office assistants)? What about your patients?
- Learn the correct methodology for testing change on a small scale. Small-scale testing is the safest and quickest way to gain knowledge about improving a system. More to come in future chapters.

The skill sets we will discuss, especially those surrounding problem solving, can be used to improve all sorts of things – from how to deliver great health care to how to deliver Chinese take out. There is no limit, and with six you get egg roll.

References

1. Institute of Medicine (US) Committee on Quality of Health Care in America. Crossing the quality chasm: a new health system for the 21st century. Washington DC: National Academy Press; 2001.
2. Nolan TW. Understanding medical systems. Ann Intern Med. 1998;128:293–8.
3. Berwick DM. A primer on leading the improvement of systems. BMJ. 1996;312(7031): 619–22.
4. Huber TP. Presentation to CCHA/CCS. http://www.dhcs.ca.gov/provgovpart/initiatives/nqi/Documents/MicroSysHC.ppt.

Chapter 6
Problem Solving

Eric D. Newman

Keywords Problem solving • Systems of care • Innovative thinking • Eight disciplines • PDCA • Define the problem • Analyze the problem • Develop some solutions • Fishbone

> *"Which Damn Button Do I Push on the Remote?" Of course, I embellish a little. My wife Laurie would never curse.*
> *In our home, we have your typical Y chromosome-induced mangle and tangle of electronic devices – digital receiver systems, house-wide music intranet, 7 speakers balanced for perfect 3D sound distribution (including a subwoofer that will loosen your neighbor's fillings), gaming boxes, digital recorders, high-def DVD players, internet streaming, flame throwers – all eventually terminating in a device traditionally known as a TV set (1080P of course). All my wife wants to do is watch HGTV (the Home & Garden Television Channel).*
> *So I tell her it's easy – take remote A and push these 3 buttons in sequence, shake remote B to wake it up (yawn) then make sure the slider is set to "TV/VCR" and push it twice (unless the previous device watched was a DVD, then just once), take the sound distribution remote and make sure it knows it's a sound distribution remote (talking to it will not accomplish this task), and push buttons 3, 4, and 6 if the broadcast is in Dolby Digital otherwise just push button 1, click your heels and say "there's no place like Danville", and voila – HGTV (although sometimes it's Fox News).*
> *She picks up one of the remotes (any one will of course do), pushes several buttons in random sequence, finds herself in the middle of a Halo battlefield, yells at me (again), then feeds several of the remotes to our dog Cooper.*

E.D. Newman, MD (✉)
Department of Rheumatology, Clinical Innovations, Division of Medicine,
Geisinger Health System, Danville, PA, USA
e-mail: arthman@aol.com

J.T. Harrington and E.D. Newman (eds.), *Great Health Care: Making It Happen*,
DOI 10.1007/978-1-4614-1198-7_6, © Springer Science+Business Media, LLC 2012

Neither of us have successfully solved the problem of watching HGTV. My solution was overly complex, and thus highly unreliable. Kind of reminds you of trying to get a follow-up appointment with your physician (call office, put on hold, push buttons 3,2,7,9 in sequence, lie that you are actually calling from a doctor's office, be put on hold again but this time with elevator music, get disconnected, call back, repeat sequence, get human, who needs to get other human, who will get right back to you).
Laurie's solution was much simpler and more elegant – but did not accomplish the task at hand (unless you're Cooper). Both of us jumped to the solution, without first understanding the problem. Keep reading – not only will you gain skills and powers enabling you to solve problems at a single bound, but at the end you will also see how to effectively unravel the HGTV Gordian Knot.

                                                                              Eric D. Newman

Life is a series of problems needing to be solved – some of them small (how do I get my socks to match) and some of them large (how do we effectively and efficiently deliver care to patients with diabetes, congestive heart failure, and severe arthritis). Fortunately, Shewart, Deming, and Ishikawa will help us. More about them later.

I want to spend a moment talking about physicians and problem solving. Let's start with my ilk – rheumatologists. We as a breed pride ourselves in our diagnostic problem-solving skills. We can take an exceedingly complex case, and in a matter of nanoseconds create a virtual differential diagnosis, accompanied by likely probabilities, a series of initial evaluations, and even the next 27 steps in workup including a dizzying array of weird and wonderful laboratory tests that follow a intense patient interrogation and a "no crevice unturned" physician examination. Point of fact, we do a really good job at it. As long as we are talking about one doc, and one patient.

The problem lies in that we have already in our head jumped to the solution. And if we apply that same thinking to solving problems in systems of care, we will assuredly make the wrong decisions. Effective problem solving in complex systems requires a rote series of steps, in order – *one of the last steps* being testing a solution. And the good news is once you learn these skills, you can apply them to an entire array of life's problems.

As a first step, I have a few painful truths for physician and administrative leaders to consider (Fig. 6.1):

- Your view from your vantage is skewed and may be wrong
- You are not an island unto yourself
- Your staff has better ideas than you do
- You don't understand what you don't measure
- Complaining is easy – change is hard

However, don't break out the hemlock yet. You can learn this and you can do this. We will begin with the 50,000 foot view (innovation) and then come down to ground level (problem solving). Let's proceed.

Your view from your vantage is skewed and may be wrong
- What do you see?
    - The patient didn't show up or call to cancel – it's the patient's fault so I will send them a bill for wasting my time
    - The Primary Care Physician (PCP) hasn't sent me any info on a new patient – it's the PCPs fault – I will bad mouth them in front of the patient
    - I can't get the nurse to prepare me an injection when I need it – I need to hire another nurse
- What is the truth?
    - The patient was never contacted about the appointment
    - The PCP's office can't get through on your fax line
    - Injection supplies not available where they are needed
- Pearl - Don't assume that what you see is necessarily the truth, and don't create a solution until you have fully analyzed the problem

You are not an island unto yourself
- We all work in a system, connected to other systems
- Systems are a set of interdependent variables that work together to achieve a common goal
- Systems are unruly
- Pearl – if you perturb your system, the upstream and downstream effects may be unpredictable. This is one reason to try "small scale tests of change"

Your staff has better ideas than you do
- Your patients also have better ideas than you do
- Create a team - include your support staff – maybe a patient
- Pearl – Empower your staff to solve problems and reward them for doing so

You don't understand what you don't measure
- Assuming your business is
    - To take excellent care of your patients
    - To provide excellent service to your referring docs
    - To have a life
- How can you run your business if you
    - Don't measure the quality you deliver?
    - Don't measure the service you provide?
    - Get home at 9pm because there is "so much work to do"?
- Pearl – Measure, measure, measure. You will be surprised at what you find, and you will be able to quantify your success as you succeed

Complaining is easy – change is hard
- There will always be resistors. Fire them, retire them, or at least ignore them
- There is an investment in time and energy that is required to effect change – it is well worth it
- Pearl - start small, pick low-hanging fruit to learn the methodology, align incentives, celebrate your successes

Fig. 6.1 A few painful truths

Innovative Thinking

Where do you spend your time – in crisis mode, in redesigning to make things better, or working on innovative projects? Most of us exist in "crisis mode" – stamping out the fires of today, leaving us no time for planning and horizon thinking. Some of us have the opportunity to work redesigning our way of care. A few of us have the extraordinary opportunity of doing innovative work.

Innovative thinking can be divided into three basic categories – viewing things differently, challenging the old way of thinking, and assuming the impossible. Let's look at an example of each category. Dean Kamen viewed transportation differently. Instead of focusing on technology to go longer distances faster, he instead focused on going shorter distances more efficiently. His invention, the Segway®, has improved the efficiency of transportation in many different sectors, including tourism, large manufacturing plants, the police force, and those individuals with walking disabilities [1].

Challenging the old way of thinking often involves turning the usual pathway 180°. In total joint replacement, the usual paradigm is education, operation, then rehabilitation. By turning this 180° and beginning with rehabilitation (termed "prehabilitation"), patient outcomes can improve [2].

Assuming the impossible is my favorite type of innovative thinking. When faced with the problem of what to do if a heart stops beating, the medical profession and society's response was to create an emergency medical system that would transport these patients to care sooner and to train vast numbers of lay people to try and keep patients alive until more definitive care could be rendered by trained personnel (basic life support – BLS). But what if you asked a 5 year old the same question – "What would you do if the heart stops beating?" The child might reply "Well, why not let the heart start itself?" By assuming the impossible, this simple reframing of the problem led to the development of the implantable defibrillator and the automatic external defibrillator – the latter device now incorporated directly into (BLS) training and available in many public locations [3].

Problem Solving

In the business world and beyond, there are many methodologies which touch on either problem solving or improving efficiency – Eight Disciplines, Six-Sigma, PDCA to name a few (Table 6.1). While primarily designed for improving quality and efficiency in manufacturing, pieces and parts can be successfully adapted for use in healthcare problem solving and redesign.

Problem solving, fortunately, is quite easy if you follow set of linear steps and do not skip any steps [4]. An analogy for healthcare providers is that problem solving is like doing a procedure – you follow a certain set of steps in order. You would never, for example, do a procedure first, and *then* do your sterile preparation.

Problem solving is no different. Why would you implement a solution before fully understanding the problem? How many times have each of us been on a committee

Table 6.1 Common problem-solving methodologies

Eight Disciplines	Six-Sigma	PDCA
Use a team approach	Define	Plan
Describe the problem	Measure	Do
Contain the problem	Analyze	Check
Identify/define/verify root causes	Improve	Act
Choose corrective actions	Control	
Implement/validate corrective actions		
Prevent recurrence		
Reward the team		

where a problem is presented, and immediately the committee begins to debate the best solution. Doctors are backed up so we will hire more doctors. Tests are too expensive so we will develop an impenetrable wall of preapproval red tape. Patients don't show up for visits we give them so we will start charging them for no-shows. All real-life solutions. None actually solve the problem with which they were supposedly associated. Oops – guess we didn't understand the problem.

I would propose a set of problem-solving steps that combines qualities of Eight Disciplines and PDCA. Short enough that it's easy to remember. Robust enough that it gets the job done:

- Define the problem
- Analyze the problem
- Develop some solutions
- Test a solution
- Measure the results of testing
- Reassess, retest, and remeasure

The remainder of this chapter will explore the first three bullet points. The next chapter (testing and implementing solutions) will focus on the second three bullet points.

"Defining the problem" is a commonly missed but very important first step. A properly defined problem has three features: (1) it is within your sphere of control, (2) you do not assume the cause, and (3) you do not have a solution in mind. For example, here is a poor way of framing a problem – "If we only had enough physicians our patient backlog would be fixed." First, this statement assumes that the reason for the backlog is not enough physicians. Second, it already provides the solution – simply hire more physicians. A better framing of the problem would be "We cannot see our patients in a timely fashion." In this statement, you did not assume you knew the reason for the backlog, and you broadened your scope to include more potential solutions – ones that are less costly and more likely to solve the problem – template management, simplification of scheduling rules, standardization of visit types, preappointment management, etc.

Once the problem has been defined, it then needs to be analyzed. There are several methodologies for doing this, commonly falling under a broader umbrella of "root-cause analysis." One of the more painful approaches (perhaps better termed root-canal analysis) is known as a causal tree. A tree structure is used to link cause/effect branches. This technique can be helpful for sentinel safety events that happen in a hospital.

Another analysis technique, somewhat easier to use, is known as the "5 whys." Sakichi Toyoda of the Toyota Motor Corporation originally developed this technique as part of Toyota's evolving strategy to improve manufacturing reliability. To do a "5 whys" analysis, you simply ask the question why five times and the root cause spits out at the bottom. Well sort of. Here is a healthcare example:

- A drug-induced blood abnormality was missed. Why?
- The ordering physician did not see the test result. Why?
- The office never received the report. Why?
- The fax machine was not operating properly. Why?
- No one was assigned to check the status of the machine. Why?
- The secretaries were busy with other duties. Root cause – the task of making sure the fax machine was working was not deemed important and hence unassigned.

A third problem analysis technique is known as a fishbone diagram. I find a fishbone diagram to be more intuitive and easier to understand. Fishbone diagrams are also known as "cause and effect" or Ishikawa diagrams. Kaoru Ishikawa developed the idea to improve production in the Kawasaki Shipyards in Japan over 40 years ago. A fishbone diagram is a picture of the factors thought to produce a certain result (main spine), with arrows representing contributing factors, which could produce this result pointing to the main spine. Figure 6.2 shows a sample fishbone diagram for appointment delays, with the main contributing categories of people, equipment, materials, and process.

Now that we have defined our problem and analyzed our problem, it is time to develop some solutions. Solution development often involves two steps: a brainstorming session followed by a prioritization session.

Brainstorming involves getting a large group of participants together to generate a long list of potential solutions. Everyone with "skin in the game" needs to be there. Someone serves as the session leader and someone else serves as a scribe. No one is criticized for his or her contributions, everyone participates, and lots of solutions with exaggerated ideas are encouraged. A healthy productive brainstorming session results in dozens of weird, whacky, and wonderful solutions magic marked up on easel tear-off sheets strewn around the room.

Prioritization involves a much smaller, more somber (and perhaps sober) decision-making group. This group prioritizes the long list of brainstorming solutions, focusing on ease of implementation and potential impact as guiding principles.

To recap, we have defined our problem, analyzed our problem, and developed some solutions. The next chapter will discuss how we might test a solution, measure the results, and reassess, remeasure, and retest. Before doing so, let's take the remote control fiasco at the chapter's beginning and apply our newly gained problem-solving knowledge:

- Define the problem – Inability to easily and reliably watch HGTV
- Analyze the problem – Contributing factors include multiple remotes, complex button choices, ill-defined processes for equipment startup, and a hungry dog

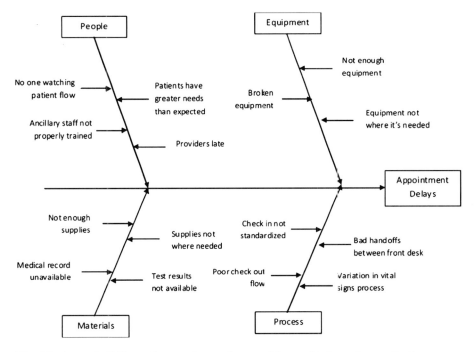

Fig. 6.2 A sample fishbone diagram for appointment delays, with the main contributing categories of people, equipment, materials, and process

- Develop some solutions – (1) replace the seven remotes with a single universal remote that allows programming a process ("I want to watch HGTV") with a single button press. (2) Feed the dog something more nutritious. (3) Buy a 152 in. 3D plasma TV (we did say that exaggerated ideas were welcome, did we not?)

Unfortunately, the prioritization committee shot down solution 3. Thus, it is with sadness that I ask you to turn to the next chapter.

References

1. Sawatzky B, Denison I, Tawashy A. The Segway for people with disabilities: meeting clients' mobility goals. Am J Phys Med Rehabil. 2009;88:484–90.
2. Jaggers JR, Simpson CD, Frost KL, et al. Prehabilitation before knee arthroplasty increases post-surgical function: a case study. J Strength Cond Res. 2007;21:632–4.
3. American Heart Association. Part 4: adult basic life support. Circulation. 2005;112:IV-19–34.
4. Harrington JT, Newman ED. Redesigning the care of rheumatic diseases at the practice and system levels: a two part article – part 1 – practice level process improvement (redesign 101). Clin Exp Rheumatol. 2007;25 Suppl 47:S55–63.

Chapter 7
Testing and Implementing Solutions

Eric D. Newman

Keywords Testing solutions • Implementing solutions • PDSA • Shewhart • Deming • Access • Pre-appointment management • Advanced access • Backlog

PDSA and IMHO
I love initialisms. An initialism is a group of letters used as an abbreviation, such as BBC – British Broadcasting Corporation. PDSA, our tool du jour for effecting change, is an initialism for "Plan-Do-Study-Act". But sometimes the same set of letters can mean different things. Doing a Google search on PDSA for example gives you "Plan-Do-Study-Act" as the 2nd hit – the 1st hit is "Platelet Disorder Support Association". Hit #7 yield's "People's Dispensary for Sick Animals". If you keep searching, you will also find .....
Persistent Data Storage Architecture
Parallel Distributed Sample Acquisition
Paid Scientific Associate
Peroxy-Disulfuric Acid
Player Development Soccer Academy
(and of course) Pacific Dolphin Swim Association
So the truth is in the ear and tongue of the beholder. Hence my embarrassing IMHO story. This story is true – you just can't make this stuff up.
About 10 years ago, I was working with some nice folks at the PA State Health Department on an osteoporosis project. We had never met one another, and much of our discourse and work was done by email. Because some of our work was eminence-based rather than evidence-based, I would begin these emails with IMHO. Most of you with kids between 12 and 22 would

E.D. Newman, MD (✉)
Department of Rheumatology, Clinical Innovations, Division of Medicine,
Geisinger Health System, Danville, PA, USA
e-mail: arthman@aol.com

J.T. Harrington and E.D. Newman (eds.), *Great Health Care: Making It Happen*,
DOI 10.1007/978-1-4614-1198-7_7, © Springer Science+Business Media, LLC 2012

recognize this as a common texting initialism (In My Humble Opinion).
This email trail went on for a number of months, until we all met at a meeting. We discussed our nice conversations together until one of the health department workers sheepishly raised a question. "Dr. Newman, you know those emails you have been sending us?" "Yes of course", I replied. "Well", she said, "we have a question for you". Why do you always call yourself a "ho" in the beginning? Is there something we should know? IMHO, in their brains, became "I'm a ho". Which is slang for the world's oldest profession. And no, I'm not.
                                                                                IMNATAHO Eric D. Newman.

In the last chapter, we discussed Kaoru Ishikawa, the father of the fishbone "cause and effect" diagram. Let's spend a few sentences on our next two heroes – Shewhart and Deming – the fathers of the Pacific Dolphin Swim Association (err, the Plan-Do-Study Act cycle).

Walter A. Shewhart was a physicist, engineer, and statistician. He was also known as the father of quality control, an area of expertise that he developed at Bell Labs during the 1930s. Dr. Shewhart conceived of the Shewhart cycle, also termed PDCA – plan-do-check-act. W. Edwards Deming, professor and statistician, took Shewhart's thoughts and recrafted it as the Deming Cycle (PDSA – plan-do-study-act). He is responsible for the major innovative changes in the Japanese manufacturing process in the 1950s and beyond, leading to Japan's dominating production of high-quality products.

So who better to assist us in taking our solutions for a spin to see what works and continuously iterate until they do, than Drs. Shewhart and Deming?

PDSA starts with an initial cycle. In that cycle, we have four steps:

Plan – state objective, predict what will happen, develop a plan
Do – do it, record problems and observations, begin data analysis
Study – complete data analysis, compare to predictions, summarize
Act – what are the modifications, what happens next cycle?

PDSA cycles are stacked on top of one another – Cycle 1, Cycle 2, Cycle 4 (just making sure you are paying attention). Most projects require a number of cycles before the process is honed and working at the level desired.

It is very important not to plan the next cycle until the proceeding cycle is completed and the results analyzed. Otherwise you have broken the cardinal rule of not proposing solutions until you have fully analyzed the problem. Or in lay terms, keep an open mind. The process of discovery using this technique often leads to unexpected solutions. Process redesign work is often counterintuitive – something that simply should not work (based on our own innate biases and erroneous assumptions) works just fine, or in a way we would not have expected. If this bothers your psyche and causes you brain freeze, take a breath. When you learn to embrace this concept, you will be able to move mountains, grasshopper.

There is no such thing as a problem too small to be solved by PDSA methodology. Let me take an example of some of our earliest work in our Rheumatology Clinic.

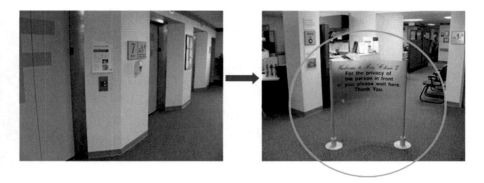

Fig. 7.1 Solving the elevatoritis conundrum

Our department suffers from a severe case of "elevatoritis". The Merck Manual defines "elevatoritis" as …

> a typical old building clinic disease, where the elevator and the front desk are built in close proximity. The elevator will paroxysmally open and spew out a dozen patients on top of the front check-in desk. The resultant symptoms including overcrowding, pushing and shoving to jockey to the front of the crowd, and loss of confidentiality as the hard of hearing are asked 300 Government-sponsored questions of little value at a high enough volume to be heard three floors below. Proposed treatments include the cone of silence, and early retirement.

A problem ripe for solving. After going through the problem-solving process, we proposed some solutions to test:

Cycle 1 – setup some strings of high intensity blinking lights to point patients in the correct direction to line up. Result – strobotic effect with petit mal seizures.

Cycle 2 – setup stanchions and ropes to cordon patients off, a la Hollywood's red carpet entrance. Results – tripping and falling, comingling of canes and walkers. Not a pretty sight.

Back to the drawing board. After speaking with one of my coworkers (see section on teaming), our fellowship administrative assistant who always likes to think outside of the box, we went back and reexamined our priorities. What were we looking for? We wanted something readable, simple, and inviting. We wanted to divert, but not obstruct. The result ….

Cycle 3 – a flexible see-through floor standing sign with large font and a friendly message (Fig. 7.1). It worked perfectly and has since been adopted by many other clinics in our healthcare system.

PDSA Healthcare Example

The above example is "small and funny." Let's look at "small and powerful." Here is a quick PDSA designed to address "no-show" rate – how can we decrease the number of patients who fail to show up for their clinic visit, so more patients can be seen (improving access) and less revenue is lost (improving profitability in this widget world of reimbursement).

Cycle 1: Improve "no-show" rate

Plan

- Call all scheduled new patients during the daytime 2 days before their scheduled visit

Do

- For 2 weeks
- Call all scheduled news 48 h before appointment
- Monitor whether patient reached (human, *LMAM, nada) and work effort (minutes per appointment)

Study

- Eighty patients called, 50% reached in person
- No-show rate higher if human not reached (LMAM plus nada)
- Cost/appointment call = $1.00 × 80 patients = $80
- 6 "no-shows" averted and filled with other patients (6 × $200/consult = $1,200)
- Net additional revenue = $1,200 − $80 = $1120 per 2 weeks = $29,120/year

Act

- For Cycle 2 – call at night to see if yield is better
- For Cycle 3 – capture preferred contact time and phone number to reach to see if reaching a human increases yield

Hmmm, let's see. Two-week study, cost basically nothing to test, used existing staff, resulted in improved access and financial performance. And this was just the first cycle!

(On soapbox) Imagine if we tried doing the same project, but making it a formal research study? It would require a sizable grant, there would have to be randomization to several different arms, someone would have to swallow a placebo capsule, it would take 3 years to accomplish, several statisticians might be hurt in the process, and it is likely the result would not be effective, as the solution was likely conceived without a careful analysis of the problem. The conclusion – "more research is needed." On to the next grant. If you were the arthritis patient waiting in pain to see the specialist, which methodology would you choose? Science is often best addressed with the scientific method. Redesign is often best addressed with problem-solving industrial-based methodology. The two can coexist happily, and each has its place. More to come in Part V (Off soapbox).

---

*LMAM, an initialism. pronounced "elmam," stands for Left Message on Answering Machine.

Now, on to more PDSA for fun and profit. We will review a few real-life examples of how powerful this methodology can be.

PDSA in Action: Improving Access to Care

Very few places in the USA can claim they have excellent access. Not surprising – we have complex appointment systems, arcane procedures, rules inflicted by physicians who can only see patients with disease "x" on Tuesday afternoons (between 1:00 and 2:20). In essence, our typical referral process is designed perfectly to achieve the result it gets. Access excellence is a bit of an oxymoron, like jumbo shrimp, great depression, even odds, and liquid gas (thanks Cooper).

Here are two access success stories – preappointment management and advanced access in specialty care. Each project attacked the same problem in a different fashion, each produced successful, sustainable, and scalable improvement.

Preappointment Management

The traditional referral process to a specialist takes a population of patients at varying degrees of risk who are referred by their primary care (physician, provider, site, medical home). This process has the following problems:

- Visit-dependent, patient-driven
- High variation, duplication, waste, and cost
- Poorly defined processes/roles roles
- Population at risk not identified and treated
- Severe cases not matched with expertise

Preappointment management [1] tries to solve these problems by accomplishing the following tasks:

- Population is defined and registered
- Care process is planned
- Provider role is defined
- Provider and patient are educated
- Measures/CQI techniques are included

Preappointment management involves reviewing of prior medical records and other pertinent information by the consultant physician before an appointment is scheduled in order to determine the most appropriate care plan for each patient. The end result is one of four outcomes:

1. Urgent, long, or short appointment
2. Alternative specialty consultation
3. Continue with referring physician
4. No consultation

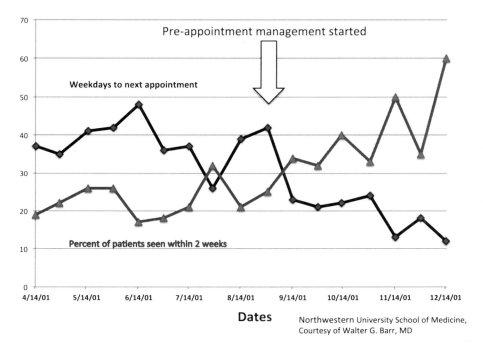

Fig. 7.2 Impact of preappointment management on patient access to rheumatology consultation

Dr. Harrington's original work in this area involved 279 referred patients. After implementing preappointment management using PDSA methodology, it was determined that 41% of the referrals did not require a specialty assessment. Over time, not only did access to care improve, but also the process resulted in primary care referring a greater portion of patients who *did* need specialty assessment over time. That is, one of the side benefits was provider education in the context of their decision-making that resulted in a sustained change in behavior. This new process of care delivery truly helped to get the right patient the right care at the right time.

Instead of presenting Dr. Harrington's results, I would like to show those of our friend and colleague, the late Dr. Walter Barr (Fig. 7.2). Dr. Barr learned the technique from Dr. Harrington and implemented the new care process at a different academic institution. Within 3 months of instituting preappointment management, the percent of new patients seen within 2 weeks rose from 23 to 60%. Additionally, the number of days to the third available appointment (a standard measure of access) fell from about 40 days to less than 20 days. These results are illustrative for three reasons. First, the results are so dramatic that no formal statistical evaluation would be needed to claim success. Second, the results show scalability – the technique worked successfully at a completely different place and environment than Dr. Harrington's work. Third, it demonstrates the importance of a provider champion to lead the way.

Advanced Access

It was February of 2001 when we began our journey of improving access to care [2]. I remember this date palpably, because at the same time we were redesigning our entire care delivery process within our department we were also "going live" on implementing our health system's electronic health record. The best analogy I can give is that it was like getting an upper and lower endoscopy, simultaneously, without propofol.

Our process of access redesign was based on the Institute for Healthcare Improvement's IDCOP program (Idealized Design for the Clinical Office Practice – another initialism!). At that time, almost all of the work was being performed in the primary care arena – the process had not been tested on the specialty side. Our department was asked (told?) to take a leap of faith – that the process could be morphed into something that would work on the specialty side. We would be the first to try. And so began a decade-long journey of discovery and change and adventure.

Our PDSA-based redesign involved four basic methodological steps:

Deal with the backlog

- Eliminate "bad backlog" (overdue patients)
- Measure "good backlog" (patients who need to be seen in the future) using capacity/demand analysis techniques

Create advanced access

- Simplify templates and remove the rules (create truth in scheduling)
- Create advanced access slots frozen in time and space (based on capacity/demand analysis)
- Open slots 5 days ahead (do not use until then!)

Retool follow-up appointment process

- ≤3 months – patient gets convenient appointment
- >3 months – patient gets reminder card and placed on follow-up list – scheduled close-in to when appointment is due. Patient asked to call us based on card. If they forget, we call them. (Why delay scheduling distant future appointments? Because the amount of rework (cancels and reschedules) for a 1-year follow-up is HUGE – Remember SYSTEMS!!!)

Develop primary care-specialist protocols

- Knee osteoarthritis (OA) referral effectiveness

  * To reduce rheumatology referrals for uncomplicated OA cases
  * Use when PCP requests rheum knee OA referral (EHR)

- Availability by text pager for referring provider calls

  * Respect systems (a PCP has 5 min with a patient)

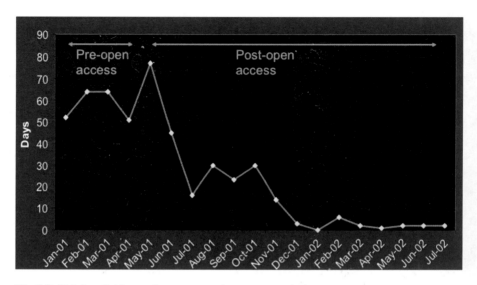

Fig. 7.3 Third available appointment pre and postaccess redesign

* If 5 min on the phone saves $1,000 in workup or an unneeded new referral, it's better care

Our results were equally dramatic (Fig. 7.3). In addition to a reduction in third available appointment (industry standard method for assessing access), our percent cancelations dropped by 50%, patient satisfaction improved significantly (we did have a "p value" for this one), referral effectiveness showed a decrease in new knee OA referrals by 7% while simultaneously increasing new referrals for rheumatoid arthritis (our goal) by 50%, and net revenue improved by $163,000 for the year.

Our project has in addition demonstrated the concept of sustainability. Over the past 10 years, through changes in providers and other team members, new regulations, and other demands of our time, we have continued to tweak our access design process. We measure, monitor, adjust, and adapt. Our excellence in access has been maintained – at the time of this writing, our "no-show" rate is 2.1%, our schedule fill rate is at ~100%, and our third available appointment is less than 1 week.

In addition to improving delivery of care for those that we serve (patients with rheumatic disease), this process has served us well in other aspects – successfully developing programs of care with our primary care colleagues, performing research and quality improvement projects, and the ability to request and receive system resources to continue our work. This last point is worth emphasizing – rheumatologists often consider themselves the "Rodney Dangerfield" specialists – we get no respect. Our ability to demonstrate success in this and other similar redesign projects resulted in a heightened level of confidence that resources spent in our area would likely result in some positive outcome. Everyone wins – patients, primary care, specialty care, administration.

We hope we have been able to show you that problem solving and redesigning healthcare delivery is do-able and rewarding. Here are a few ingredients for success that should resonate:

- Remember the painful truths!
- Learn the methodology
- Form a redesign team and meet regularly
- Teach them what we have just taught you
- Go through the process with a small problem
- Fail and learn and try again
- Celebrate your success and share it with others

To help tie *"Part II"* all together, I will leave you with some of my favorite problem-solving and redesign quotes:

The significant problems we face cannot be solved at the same level of thinking we were at when we created them

Albert Einstein

I have not failed 700 times. I have not failed once. I have succeeded in proving that those 700 ways will not work. When I have eliminated the ways that will not work, I will find the way that will work

Thomas Edison

Do, or do not. There is no try

Master Jedi Yoda

A child of five could understand this. Fetch me a child of five

Groucho Marx

And my favorite ....

"If toast always lands butter-side down, and cats always land on their feet, what happens if you strap toast on the back of a cat and drop it?"

Steven Wright

Sometimes you just have to go out there and do it.

References

1. Harrington JT, Walsh MB. Pre-appointment management of new patient referrals in rheumatology: a key strategy for improving health care delivery. Arthritis Rheum. 2001;45(3): 295–300.
2. Newman ED, Harrington TM, Olenginski TP, Perruquet JL, McKinley K. "The rheumatologist can see you now": Successful implementation of an advanced access model in a rheumatology practice. Arthritis Rheum. 2004;51:253–7.

Part III
Managing Chronic Disease: You Can't Do Things Differently Until You See Things Differently

Eric D. Newman

The ultimate concrete thinkers are kids. They know what they hear, and they then know what they know. No wiggle room for interpretation. One brief example for you. My son Nathaniel (then 5) approached me one morning very upset about Cassie (our 1 year-old golden retriever). "Is Cassie ok?" "Yes" I replied, somewhat perplexed. "But is she ok??" "Yes Nathaniel, Cassie is just fine." At this point, Nathaniel's voice started to quiver. "But dad, is Cassie really alright?" I asked him to tell me what was wrong. Between near sobs, he replied, "I heard you tell mom that Cassie was barking her head off." Doesn't get more concrete than that!

This part is all about managing – managing complexity, information, process, outcome, people, and reimbursement. The chapters herein will review the challenges we face, and some fresh ideas and solutions to consider. Inherent in that consideration is a willingness to think, and eventually act, outside of what might be your comfort zone today. You cannot do things differently until you see things differently. Maybe start by developing some flexibility – moving beyond the concrete thinking that holds us back.

So watch what you say. Watch what you do. And don't try to manage another thing in life until you read this part.

E.D. Newman, MD
Department of Rheumatology, Clinical Innovations,
Division of Medicine, Geisinger Medical Center,
Danville, PA, USA

Chapter 8
Managing Complex Processes: Making Order Out of Chaos

J. Timothy Harrington

Keywords Complex processes • Managing • Health systems • High performance • Culture • Performance excellence • Goals • Incentives • Measurement

In the 1970s, I served as internal medicine clerkship coordinator at the University of Texas Health Sciences Center in San Antonio. Medical students had been starting the 3rd year clerkship primed with knowledge, a long medical history and physical exam outline, and a stethoscope. They had no idea how to function in the clinical environment. They were expected to learn these skills on their own, or not at all.

We developed a "Clinical Logic and Processes" course at the end of the second preclinical year. We taught the clinicians-to-be how to create a problem list, to write a standardized set of orders, and to present a summary of a patient's data and problems. They also watched twelve videotapes of experienced clinicians performing comprehensive histories and physical exams – learning by patterning, or see-one-do-one-teach-one in the classroom. The new clerks hit the deck running.

At their Senior Skits two years later, my first class satirized me as an obsessive-compulsive super market checker who demanded that they organize their purchases just so on the counter and present them to me in standardized language. "No! Vegetables first or you go to the back of the queue!" They actually got it!

J. Timothy Harrington

One of the fundamental opportunities for a health system is to standardize care processes and to accelerate learning among the health system organization for adoption of best practices (Julie Yonek, Stephen Hines, and Maulik Joshi, 2010 [1]).

J.T. Harrington, MD (✉)
Division of Rheumatology, University of Wisconsin School of Medicine
and Public Health, Madison, WI, USA
e-mail: timharrington@charter.net

J.T. Harrington and E.D. Newman (eds.), *Great Health Care: Making It Happen*,
DOI 10.1007/978-1-4614-1198-7_8, © Springer Science+Business Media, LLC 2012

*In 1910, in his recommendations for reforming medical
education, Abraham Flexner responded to what he deemed to
be the "public interest." Now, 100 years later, to respond to the
current needs of society, the education of physicians must once
again change. In addition to understanding the biologic basis of
health and disease, and mastering technical skills for treating
individual patients, physicians will need to learn to navigate in
and continually improve complex systems in order to improve
the health of the patients and communities they serve.*

Donald M. Berwick and Jonathan Finkelstein, 2010 [2]

Complex processes and systems are inherently unruly, as already discussed in
Part II. Individuals and organizations that exist in such environments must either
manage complexity, or their performance will be degraded by it. The complexity of
health care has exploded in the last 50-plus years, as the Institute of Medicine has
documented, and as described in Part I. More often than not, performance degradation has outpaced management of complexity in the financing and delivery of health
care, leading to high costs and suboptimal results.

In 1988, Peter Drucker wrote in his Harvard Business Review essay, The Coming
of the New Organization, "Twenty years from now, the typical large business will
have half the levels of management and one third the managers of its counterpart
today. Work will be done by specialists brought together in task forces that cut
across traditional departments. Coordination and control will depend largely on
employees' willingness to discipline themselves. Behind these changes lies information technology."

Well, 20 years have gone by, and health care is a large business, but has yet to be
transformed in the ways Peter Drucker predicted, even though his vision still identifies what needs to change, and generally has not.

The Emergence of High-Performing Health Systems

Fortunately, exceptional health systems have turned the tables on complexity and
degradation of performance, as described best in a recently published report by
Yonek et al from the Health Research and Education Trust [1]. These researchers
and others engaged in healthcare improvement have concluded that high performance needs to be pursued beyond the individual provider and encounter levels,
and that it can be achieved most effectively at the local and broader health system
levels. Until providers and payers standardize work around best practices and
teamwork, performance will be compromised by high variance and inefficiency. It
is futile for individual providers to do their own thing, however well motivated
they may be.

Yonek's group studied the 200 largest multihospital health systems in the United
States and used independent quality data to separate high and low performers.
Several themes emerged:

- No one type of system was associated with high performance.
- No one factor was clearly associated with high performance.
- Creating a culture of performance excellence, accountability for results, and effective leadership are the keys to success.

They next identified specific behaviors that were associated with high performance, which included:

- Establishing a system-wide strategic plan with measurable goals
- Creating alignment across the health system with goals and incentives
- Leveraging data and measurement across the organization
- Standardizing and spreading best practices across the health system

High-performing health systems beat lower performing systems in all of these categories, and system-based chronic disease management has been one of their best achievements. This study mirrors a 1990s study by Collins and Porras, reported in "Built to Last" [3]. They compared visionary companies to lower performing successful companies across a wide range of industries other than health care. Again, the former were distinguished by cultures of performance excellence, accountability for results, and effective leadership. In fact, much of what has been used to achieve healthcare transformation has been borrowed from other industries. For these reasons, we should continue learning from high-performing organizations inside and outside of the health system, and both of these studies should be read by anyone who is serious about redesigning health care.

So how do we begin to deal with the complexity in health care, given that most providers exist currently in small, weakly coordinated single specialty practices that do not often measure performance, or only measure what they can do individually, and get paid well without measuring anything but revenues and expenses. To begin, we must:

- Acknowledge the need to improve and to measure
- Work to standardize those processes we use personally, and those we share with our partners within our practice
- Adopt and continuously improve information management processes and tools
- Learn quality improvement and clinical measurement methods
- Advocate for interdisciplinary care of patients with chronic diseases in our own practice and local healthcare environment
- Seek the support of our partners, the other colleagues that share the care of our patients, and our health system leaders

A couple of cautions are in order. First, if we do these things, we are likely to find that some of our colleagues will object, because they are wedded to individuality and value their entitlement to do things their own way. Many medical practices are built around honoring these attitudes. We call this the "free range chicken" model, in which practices are condominiums, sharing little more than some of their expenses and a call schedule. Variance may go unrecognized by physicians except when we cross-cover our vacationing partners. But ask the office staff what they think, as they try to accommodate this variance. Our second caution: sooner or later the simplest change, however positive in isolation, will begin to perturb the broader practice and system. These effects will be better accepted if others are made aware in advance, and if system leaders are asked for their support early on.

On the other hand, if you exist in one of those exceptional high-performing health systems, consider yourself fortunate, but also recognize your responsibilities to be informed and to get involved. Working for these higher purposes is personally transforming. Or if you are a nonadopter by nature, at least get out of others' way, or perhaps consider another profession!

Our improvement champions' stories in Part IV will provide examples of how to build new processes that triumph over the complexity inherent in managing populations of chronic disease patients. These champions are the ones who in each case provided the spark and exercised the necessary persistence, but their successes depended on building provider teams with clearly defined roles, measuring processes and outcomes, continuously improving and standardizing work, and working across specialties to manage the hand-offs.

Two brief examples from my personal experience also illustrate how we have developed high performance care, one within my practice and the other in our health system.

Example 1 – Practice redesign. In 2004, I decided to begin a practice improvement project to redesign the care of my patients with rheumatoid arthritis (RA). I informed my partners that I would be doing this and offered to share any successes I achieved with them. My nurse coordinator and I began by developing a practice registry of all of my RA patients. Next, we tested and implemented a standardized data collection process borrowed from the Consortium of Rheumatology Researchers of North America, Inc. (CORRONA), including both patient and physician data questionnaires, so we were collecting the same information at each visit. We had to modify our visit workflow and create different roles for patients, nursing, and me to collect this information efficiently.

Standardized data facilitated more efficient charting, more dependable documentation for billing, quantitative measurement of disease activity, and better disease outcomes. Six years later, an office visit takes me 40% less time from start to finish, not only because of standardization and efficiency, but because 80% of my RA patients now have well-controlled disease that takes less time to manage. I can estimate who will need more of my time, and who won't from the patient's questionnaire. Patients love helping me understand their problems better. In turn, I can focus on solving them [4].

Example 2 – System redesign. In 1996, one of two orthopedic spine surgeons in our group practice retired, and no replacement could be found. Their two physicians and two physician assistants (PAs) had been seeing more than 100 new consultations for back pain monthly, all comers on a first-come first-served basis. Many patients had acute self-limited pain, and less than 5% ended up having surgery. With one less physician, the wait time for a new consultation quickly extended from several weeks to over 6 months. The new patient no-show rate increased quite predictably to 40%. Instead of the right patients getting the right care at the right time, patients were getting no care at all when they needed it! My overwhelmed surgical colleague and I began a process improvement Plan-Do-Study-Act project [5].

Cycle 1: An orthopedic nurse clinician called over 200 previously scheduled new patients to determine whether they still needed care, starting with the following week's schedule, and then moving further out in time. Forty percent were either better, or had made other arrangements – no-shows in the making. She asked the rest about "red flag symptoms" that would suggest a need for urgent evaluation. If they had them, they were moved to the head of the list, usually filling slots vacated by those who no longer needed care. Then less urgent patients were also moved up into open slots.

Cycle 2: The nurse clinician then began to proactively screen all new referrals. Those with "red flags" were given an urgent appointment. Chronic back pain patients were scheduled with a rheumatologist or orthopedic PA. We discovered that 50% of referrals had acute uncomplicated low back pain and were being referred rather than being managed by their primary physician. Receptionists in our Ob-Gyn practice, the leading source of these referrals, routinely gave the Spine Orthopedic phone number to any patient who called in to be seen for low back pain.

Cycle 3: We initiated a primary care education program to teach the guidelines for back pain management, provided physician and patient teaching materials, and asked primary physicians to provide the initial care themselves. We learned that patients were often requesting these referrals, but that they were generally happy to continue primary care when assured that this was effective. Spine physical therapy was incorporated for urgent treatment of acute sciatica and for routine rehabilitation of chronic mechanical back pain. Access to care was monitored and maintained. Patient satisfaction surveys gave our management program high marks. The patients seen by the spine surgeon who received surgery increased to 30%.

Over 10 years later, we still have one spine orthopedic surgeon supported by three physician assistants, and a nurse clinician who continues our preappointment management program. Patients are happy, referring physicians are happy, and I like to say, "We just send our spine surgeon to the OR and hand him a sandwich between cases – ham and cheese, no mayo." Right patient, right care, right time, right meal.

References

1. Yonek J, Hines S, Joshi M. A guide to achieving high performance in multi- hospital health systems. Chicago, IL: Health Research & Educational Trust; March 2010.
2. Berwick DM, Finklestein JA. Preparing medical students for the continual improvement of health and health care: Abraham Flexner and the new "public interest". Acad Med. 2010;85: S56–65.
3. Collins JC, Porras JI. Built to last. New York, NY: HarperCollins; 1994.
4. Harrington JT. The uses of disease activity scoring and the physician global assessment of disease activity for managing rheumatoid arthritis in rheumatology practice. J Rheumatol. 2009;36:925–9.
5. Harrington JT, Dopf CA, Chalgren CS. Implementing guidelines for interdisciplinary care of low back pain: a critical role for pre-appointment management of specialty referrals. Jt Comm J Qual Improv. 2001;27:651–63.

Chapter 9
Managing Medical Information
(Tools, Rules, and What's Cool)

Eric D. Newman

Keywords Managing • Medical information • Weight of medical knowledge • Index medicus • Tools • Electronic health record • Luddites • Touchscreen questionnaire • PACER

The Ectopic Brain
I'm not exactly sure when I started using the term "ectopic brain". My first recollection was during medical school. The Washington Manual was considered a required resource for the wards. We used it to brush up on medical factoids moments before the ritual pimping we received from our attending physicians, who were exceedingly skilled in the Socratic method of torture. The Washington Manual was our ectopic brain – there to provide information at our fingertips – either information that we knew and needed verification, or arcane information that simply could not be remembered for longer than a single pimp.
As an aside, demonstrating once again the complexity of systems, there was a significant disconnect between the publishers of the Washington Manual (Lippincott Williams & Wilkins) and the manufacturers of medical student white coats. The Washington Manual, used by EVERY medical student, would not fit in ANY of the coat pockets!! My then girlfriend (and now wife) sewed a pocket that was specifically sized for the Washington Manual on the inside of my med student white coat. I was in intellectual heaven – my back-up brain was there for me when I needed it. Of course, as guys are want to do, this concept spread to shoving multiple other objects in various additional pockets – other reference books, reflex hammers,

E.D. Newman, MD (✉)
Department of Rheumatology, Clinical Innovations, Division of Medicine,
Geisinger Health System, Danville, PA, USA
e-mail: arthman@aol.com

stethoscopes, tuning forks, PB&J sandwiches – until I looked as
though I had hip protectors. But I digress.
The main purpose of this diatribe was to describe my best
"ectopic brain" story – and yes it's true. My undergraduate
years at Johns Hopkins were spent in fierce competition with
the next guy/gal. Everyone was premed. Everyone was driven.
Our Organic Chemistry course was the "weeder" – to weed out
those that simply were not cut out for medicine (a lousy and
blunt tool if you ask me). So everyone was hyped up for the first
major Organic Chem test.
The professor was kind enough to let us ask some questions about
the upcoming exam. "Can we bring our calculators?" "Yes",
was the reply. "Can we bring our notes?" "Yes you can", came
the less than patient reply. "Can we bring this.... bring that ...
bring some ....". Our professor's patience grew thin. Finally, in a
fit of academic rage, spittle emanating from several directions
simultaneously, he shouted "You can bring whatever you want
into the exam if you can carry it on your back, ok???!!!"
At test time, one of my classmates brought in a graduate student
strapped to his back.

Eric Newman

So many tools so little time. My dad used to say "a poor workman blames his tools." No doubt, but a corollary might be "better to be skilled with power tools than skilled with bare hands." Before we discuss the various power tools available to manage the universe of medical information, I thought it apropos to review a little history – in particular, the explosive history of medical information and the history of informational device evolution.

Most of us feel weighed down by the heavy and increasing burden of medical reading. Our inevitable failure of the struggle 'to keep up with the literature' often generates anxiety and guilt. We are all aware that the situation has worsened in the past few years, and that no respite can be expected in the future.

Durack [1]

This is a sentiment that rings true for all of us as practitioners of medicine. Of note, however, is that this quote is from 1978 – nearly a third of a century ago.

I would suggest in your copious free time that you read Dr. Durack's three page article and enjoy his wry sense of humor. The title of his work is "The Weight of Medical Knowledge," and indeed, that's exactly what he measured – the weight of the literature as represented by the *Index Medicus*. Since its inception in 1879 by Dr. John S. Billings, the *Index Medicus* has recorded (indexed) the medical literature on a yearly basis. Dr. Durack took the *Index Medicus* volumes, beginning in 1879, and weighed them in 10-year aliquots. He found a stable mass of 2 kg/year for about 60 years, followed by an exponential growth phase beginning in 1946. Between 1955 and 1977, the weight increased more than 7 times.

As a scientist, Dr. Durack was also quick to point out an inherent bias in his methodology. In later *Index Medicus* years, thinner paper was used and margins were reduced, grossly underestimating the actual increase in publications as measured

Table 9.1 Growth in publications indexed in MEDLINE	Between 1978–1985 and 1994–2001
	• 46% increase in annual MEDLINE articles
	• 272,344 articles/year to 442,756 articles/year
	• 1.88 million pages/year to 2.79 million pages per year
	• 5,174 RCTs/year to 24,724 RCTs/year

RCT = randomized clinical trials

by weight – his surrogate process measure. Unfortunately, his article lacked any statistical analysis of true outcome measures, such as medical student hernias per year. But there are amusing pictures of him demonstrating his methodological approach – standing in front of the scale, comparing 1879 (smiling) to 1974 (haggard look), bowtie and all.

So as not to skip a beat (or year), we pick up again in 1978. Druss and colleagues [2] reviewed the actual volume of publications from 1978 to 2001 using MEDLINE, the National Library of Medicine's online counterpart to the *Index Medicus*. During that interval, there were 8.1 million articles published in MEDLINE. Table 9.1 shows some journal publication facts good for a cocktail party. However, if this is the type of conversation you have at a cocktail party, please do not invite me.

Several additional observations are in order. First, over the period of observation, there was a significant shift from basic science to clinical topics. Second, there was a rise in the proportion of articles funded solely by private sources (11–27%). Finally, the National Library of Medicine estimates that it is only indexing about one quarter of the biomedical journals, demonstrating the sheer number of publications and attendant morass of information through which a diligent provider needs to sift. But do not hurry, do not scurry, we will outline ways to deal with the weight.

So let's move from this in-depth scientific review of the proliferation of medical knowledge, to my own personal journey of informational devices I acquired over the decades. As a disclaimer, the information that follows is highly biased, of questionable scientific veracity, and contains no "p" values. Enjoy.

Like many of us, it started with a slide rule. The only distinguishing feature was whether the slide rule was worn in the shirt pocket, or hung from the belt. The latter was associated with a 1.3 RR (relative risk) of getting beat up in school.

It was 1973. The first practical calculator was released to the masses – the Texas Instrument SR-10. It could perform basic math functions, was the size of a small paperback novel, and had the coolest red LED lights with squared off numbers (formed by lines intersecting only at right angles). It cost a hundred bucks, but it was well worth it to be geeked out in high school physics class.

From there, it was a series of personal computers, initially to program and play, later to do some serious work:

- 1981 – Timex Sinclair 1,000 (chicklet keys, BASIC programming language, hooked up to my black and white TV as the monitor)
- 1982 – Commodore 64 (64 kb of memory, beginning to get some productivity software)
- 1985 – Commodore Amiga (the first multitasking computer, with amazing graphics and music rendering abilities)

Then came the PDAs – personal digital assistants. I didn't jump on the palm pilot bandwagon, but instead went down the path less traveled – Pocket PCs (HP Jornada, IPAQs, and the like). These devices allowed for information to be stored and carried with you – the first practical electronic "ectopic brains." About the same time, cell phones were shrinking from the size of a brick to a svelte deck (or two) of playing cards. I remember my then young children remarking that "daddy looks like a policeman." I had my Pocket PC clipped to one hip, my cell phone clipped to another hip, and my beeper clipped to (fill in the blank). It's a wonder my pants stayed up.

Thank goodness for convergence. I now have a single device that serves as my information source and telecommunications device – my smartphone. Unfortunately, I still carry a %*&^$ beeper. But at least I don't need to add any holes in my belt anymore.

Tools

So we have established that the mass of medical information is beyond human ability to access, assess, and integrate into our neurons, and there are devices that allow us to take this information with us. But condensing information doesn't necessarily make it useful. We need tools to help us manage information – be it medical information about a condition, or medical information about a human in front of us.

Fortunately, there are many excellent internet-based tools for organizing the information available and allowing us to search for it in a meaningful fashion. Table 9.2 shows the Health Science Library clinical tools that are available to my institution's providers on our internal web.

Many of these tools are simply glorified search engines – spitting back articles of relevance in great part determined by the skill set of the searcher. Too broad a search? Get 4,357 articles about everything from artificial insemination to artificial turf. Too narrow a search? Get two articles in Mandarin about Kashin-Bek disease (look it up in your Funk & Wagnalls). Thank goodness we are fortunate enough to still have Medical Librarians, who remain one of the most service oriented personnel in the medical arena. They take your porridge that is too hot or too cold and serve it to you warm.

Table 9.2 Health sciences library clinical tools

ACS	MD consult
AccessMedicine	Natural medicines
AccessSurgery	Natural standard
Bioethics Information	NORD rare disorders
CINAHL	Nursing consult
Clinical Trials	Nursing reference center
Emergency Medical Abstracts	OVID
Harrison's Internal Medicine	Taber's Online
Health and Psychosocial Instruments	UptoDate
JBI COnNECT	Visual DX

One of more practical tools is UptoDate®, which provides not only an easy to use search engine, but information that is practical from a clinical perspective. UptoDate® combines evidence- and eminence-based medicine in just the right balance, giving clinicians helpful guidance for the types of patients they have in their office prepared by authorities on whatever the topic. It combines CME to boot and is updated often.

What about medical information for the patient in front of us? Enter the EHR – the electronic health record. A boon to improve the quality and safety of patient care? Absolutely. A panacea to cure all of our ills? Absolutely not. For the remainder of this chapter, I will explore the use of EHRs, how best to use them (rules), some of their limitations, and current and future tools that will extend the reach of electronic information management of patients and populations (what's cool).

Rules

Tuesday, Feb 13, 2001. This date may mean nothing to you, but it is indelibly etched in my brain. It was the day we went "live" on our electronic health record. Everyone remembers that day. Adapting and adjusting to an EHR is the single most awe-inspiring change event that providers will ever experience – much more of an adaption for those who practiced during the paper chart days.

Converting to using an EHR will be easiest for

- Those with computer and keyboard savvy
- Those who can change/adapt their behaviors

and will be hardest for

- Those that resist change
- Those who are Luddites*

There are significant advantages to using an EHR over the paper record. These include improvements:

- In documentation
- In safety
- In efficiency
- In population management
- In creating a culture of change

Using an EHR allows one to *document* in a consistent manner, so that the same information is found in the same way in the same location. More importantly, it is readable! If you think this is a minor issue, I would challenge any of you to pick up a paper chart and review physician notes and handwriting. Most of us took a specific course in medical school entitled "Bad Penmanship 101." I aced it. Our residents who

---

*In the nineteenth century, the Luddites were social protestors of the Industrial Revolution, destroying weaving looms – the technology of the day – in defense of weaving by hand. The term Luddite has since been used as anyone who shuns technology.

are doing retrospective chart reviews for research will sometimes come across one of my old clinic notes that they need to interpret. Several commented that they found their background knowledge of ancient hieroglyphs to be of help in that regard.

For patient *safety*, simply having a readable, dynamic, and updatable medication list that picks from a standardized database allows a source of medication truth (far removed from "I take 3 red pills, and sometimes two of the pretty blue ones"). It also provides the ability to look for potentially harmful interactions when prescribing a new medicine.

Efficiency is gained by the development of smart tools – programmed functionality that allows for easier documentation, ordering, communication, and results reviewing. For example, one can create a smart filter to review the last ten CBCs and Renal Function Panels in flowsheet form with a click of a button.

Understanding *populations* is accomplished by developing a standardized problem list and using those problems as a source of truth to develop decision support tools (e.g., who needs a flu shot, mammogram, etc). Finally, with regard to *creating a culture of change*, the process of simply going live on an EHR forces the effected individuals to change their behavior – or die a painful and horrible death by keyboard.

So why isn't everyone enamored with and actively using an EHR? While there are lots of reasons, I will focus on just two – preparation and design.

We were lucky, or maybe smart. Our institution spent an enormous amount of time preparing for go-live. Our department was challenged 6 months ahead of time to meet regularly, gain consensus on documentation and tools needed, abstract charts from the paper world to the electronic world, etc. We had excellent information technology support, before, during, and after go-live. We hit the ground running. We scaled up to the full version at a decent pace. We did it right.

Of course, we weren't the first at our institution, and the other thing we did right was learn from our mistakes, and adjust and adapt quickly. I can sum up our first EHR go-live in one word – diarrhea.

It seems the prevailing thinking at the time was that going live on an EHR should be done all at once, not piece-meal. This type of technology introduction was referred to as the "big bang" approach. Our very first primary care site to go-live used this approach. Despite the preparation, trying to do so many new tasks led the providers to do anything – *anything* – to simply get through their busy day. As primary care providers, they have 5 minutes to talk about seat belts and lasix and then the visit is over.

One of the EHR quirks is that the provider needs to associate a diagnosis with every single order – medications, labs, X-rays, return to school slips. The providers were so overwhelmed with associating diagnoses with orders that they took the path of least resistance. Every order they placed was associated with the same diagnosis –787.91. Diarrhea.

So for the next few weeks, every single patient coming into this clinic in Northeast PA left with a diagnosis of loose stools. In retrospect, I am surprised it didn't result in a CDC or USDA investigation. After that, we learned to stage the go-live process more slowly, and the outbreak of diarrhea mysteriously disappeared.

What's Cool

So you have decided to spend the money and implement an EHR. Why aren't all of your problems solved? Because most EHRs don't provide the information we need at the time we need it in the form we need it to provide optimum care.

Huh? I thought we just said that EHRs provide many tools and have many advantages over the paper record? They do, and they are a wonderful advancement. But we still have a ways to go. Future opportunities (what's cool) can be broadly divided into point-of-service opportunities (patient is in front of you) and population opportunities (between patient visits)

Point-of-service opportunities

- Assign the right task to the right team member
- Collect patient-reported information and disease outcomes
- Assemble information into actionable views

One of the common complaints is that EHRs are very provider-centric. We expect the provider to remember to order the mammograms, and the flu shot, in that same 5-min visit mentioned above. Point of fact, providers in general are highly unreliable in performing these tasks. Turns out, nurses are excellent at it.

What's cool – we turned over the tasks of addressing all alerts – "pop-ups" signaling that an event of importance needs to be done – to the nurses, with highly successful results. But it required reprogramming and restructuring of flows and roles.

EHRs do not in general come with patient questionnaire-capturing ability. Obtaining information up-front from patients not only saves considerable time, it also provides more patient-centric care. The provider is armed and ready before entering the patient's room. It helps to avoid OBTW syndrome, which commonly occurs as the provider is escorting the patient to the check out area. "Oh by the way (OBTW) I am having crushing substernal chest pain."

What's cool – we have developed a touchscreen questionnaire that the patient completes in the waiting room and integrated it into a visual display tool.

EHRs do indeed have a lot of helpful information, but that information is scattered across a myriad of tabs and subsections. We did a small PDSA project examining how long it would take for a rheumatologist to generate a very simple mental dashboard – search the EHR for the core data needed before entering a room. It averaged about 17 min! In addition, as chronic disease physicians, we want to understand patient response over time in the context of the medications we have given them. This is an impossible task with most EHRs. It would require literally reviewing every clinic note, one note at a time, and mentally assembling a patient's medication exposure over time, while simultaneously recording his or her documented functional status and disease activity.

What's cool – we developed specialized software that interfaces with the EHR, the patient, the nurse, and the provider. It's called PACER (PAtient Centric Electronic

Redesign). PACER not only pulls information from multiple disparate sources and assembles it into a set of actionable views, but also displays functional status and disease activity measures over time in the context of medication and treatment exposure. PACER also autogenerates a clinic note, creates a patient-friendly after visit summary, shines your shoes, and whistles Dixie, albeit off-key.

Population opportunities

- Develop registry functions
- Metric things other than labs
- Provide decision support

Most EHRs do not provide the ability to develop and easily use patient registries. In addition, most EHRs don't allow the capture and analysis of numeric measures that are not lab values (e.g., composite measures) or are text-based (e.g., "high risk for fracture" on DXA scan). Decision support, the ability to drive medical decision-making, is either lacking or requires extensive specialized programming.

What's cool – we have developed sophisticated methodologies for handling large amounts of data. We have created disease registries and tools for measuring disease-specific patients care gaps. We have created reports (bundles) which allow providers timely feedback of the quality of care they deliver in the context of their department, the healthcare system, and national benchmarks. Finally, we use the registry information to create visual display tools and to drive decision support – helping to close those care gaps while simultaneously measuring the effect on quality, and eventually cost.

So there you have it. Medical information is growing at such an accelerated rate that it has become far important to know where to get the answer than to actually know the answer. Optimal patient care requires actionable information that allows providers and team members to deliver the right care at the right time – whether the patient is in front of you in the clinic or at home watching reality TV. And there is a cure for diarrhea – just ask the docs in Northeast PA.

References

1. Durack DT. The weight of medical knowledge. N Engl J Med. 1978;298(14):773–5.
2. Druss BG, Marcus SC. Growth and decentralization of the medical literature: implications for evidence-based medicine. J Med Libr Assoc. 2005;93(4):499–501.

Chapter 10
Measuring Processes and Outcomes of Care

J. Timothy Harrington

Keywords Measuring • Outcomes • Processes • Zero sum game • Quality • Value • Cost • Performance measurement • Culture of measurement

You don't understand what you don't measure. Assuming your business is

- *To take excellent care of patients*
- *To provide excellent service to your referring docs*
- *To have a life, how can you run your business if you*
- *Don't measure the quality you deliver*
- *Don't measure the service you provide*
- *Get home at 9 p.m. because there's "so much work to do"*

Measure, measure, measure. You will be surprised what you find, and you will be able to quantify your success as you succeed

(From a practice redesign teaching slide, Eric D. Newman). About 5 years ago, I was giving a lecture to about 100 rheumatologists on "Redesigning Your Practice". To size up my audience, I asked, "How many of you know what the Institute of Medicine Chasm Report is?" One hand went up at the back of the room; the rest of the audience sat on theirs. So I asked him, "How did you learn about it?" He responded, "I heard your talk a year ago." Now I always ask this question, and sometimes I get 3 or 4 hands raised, often from more than 2 people. That's what I call measurable improvement!

J. Timothy Harrington

"The only way to know whether the quality of care is improving is to measure performance"

Harvey V. Fineberg, M.D., Ph.D. President, Institute of Medicine 2006 [1].

J.T. Harrington, MD (✉)
Division of Rheumatology, University of Wisconsin School of Medicine
and Public Health, Madison, WI, USA
e-mail: timharrington@charter.net

J.T. Harrington and E.D. Newman (eds.), *Great Health Care: Making It Happen*,
DOI 10.1007/978-1-4614-1198-7_10, © Springer Science+Business Media, LLC 2012

Measuring healthcare processes and the outcomes of care is surprisingly a new idea, and a chasm exists regarding the perceived need for clinical measurement between health policy experts and government planners on the one hand and the providers of care on the other. This might be considered the "second quality chasm". The train full of researchers, planners, and payers is miles down the tracks, while the train for the physicians who provide the care is just being loaded. In fact, many physicians aren't convinced that this is a train they want to ride on. As an example, Medicare has developed the Physicians Quality Reporting Initiative (PQRI) to encourage physicians to begin reporting important quality indicators, but few are participating. Doing so not only requires time and resources, but it is not part of physicians' training or self-expectations.

What Should We Be Measuring?

Let's begin by talking about what we are talking about. Regrettably, various stakeholders in the health system have adopted a variety of definitions of "quality" that often support their own self-interests. An alphabet soup of organizations has evolved which exists to generate and validate quality measures – HEDIS, NCQA, AQA, NQF, etc. They have defined a myriad of measures, largely for fragmented care processes rather than outcomes. Insurers have incorporated these into a blizzard of idiosyncratic "quality" programs. As a result, quality measurement has become one more aspect of health system dysfunction, and more hassle for physicians. Until the players agree to what healthcare "quality" and "value" mean, how can these be measured meaningfully and practically, and in ways that improve rather than interfere with healthcare delivery?

Enter Michael Porter, the Harvard economist we referred to in Section I for his portraying the US Health System as a "Zero Sum Game". His recently published perspective, "What is Value in Health Care?" and two accompanying supplements [2–4], reject most current approaches to quality measurement: "The quality movement in health care is welcomed and overdue. But today's confusion is deterring more fundamental outcome measurements."

Porter proposes that we focus on healthcare value rather than quality, as is done in other areas of our economy. "Defining and measuring value is essential to understanding the performance of any organization and driving continuous improvement. In health care, value is defined as the patient health outcomes achieved per dollar spent…It is value for the patient that is the central goal, not value for the other actors per se" (Fig. 10.1) Porter focuses on value of care, defined by outcomes for

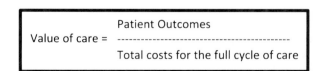

$$\text{Value of care} = \frac{\text{Patient Outcomes}}{\text{Total costs for the full cycle of care}}$$

Fig. 10.1 Value equation

patients and the total costs for the entire episode of care. This construct rejects many current approaches that consider process measures as sufficient and focus on weak predictors of "quality", such as access to care and patient satisfaction:

"Outcomes, the numerator of the value equation, refer to actual results of care in terms of patient health… The full set of outcomes, adjusted for individual patient circumstances, constitutes the quality of care for the patient…. Cost, the denominator of the equation, refers to the total costs involved in the full cycle of care for the patient's medical condition (or for his or her primary and preventive care), not just the costs involved in any one intervention or care episode. Value is increased by reducing the total costs involved in care, not necessarily minimizing the cost of individual services. To reduce cost, the best approach is often to spend more on some high-value services, frequently including preventive or other earlier-stage care, in order to reduce the cumulative cost of care over the full care cycle".

"He continues, "Value measurement in health care today is limited and highly imperfect….current organizational structure and information systems make it challenging to measure (and deliver) value. Today, measurement focuses overwhelmingly on care processes…. Compliance with evidence-based guidelines is often seen as an end in itself, without the need to measure outcomes. What is measured today, then, reflects current organizational structure and billing practices. Process measurement is useful and should continue. …a natural step in the progression of measurement, (it) should not become a sticking point or even a justification for not moving to outcome measurement. …There is no substitute for measuring actual outcomes…."

"Systematic, rigorous outcome measurement remains rare, but a growing number of examples of comprehensive outcome measurement provide evidence of its feasibility and impact…. If all the actors in health care were to embrace value as the central goal and measure value universally, the resulting improvements in health care delivery would be enormous".

The Google Earth and Ground-Level Views of Performance Measurement

Two current and discordant approaches to performance measurement need to become better integrated than at present. The first (Google Earth) is the developing of rigorous validated measures and their use by health policy researchers and government policy wonks. Their publications and position papers derived from large population databases call attention to the deficiencies and waste in health care, including chronic disease care in the US. They often end with the statement that "More research is needed," but seldom include recommendations for applying the findings to actually improve care. The second is measuring processes and outcomes within practices and local health systems – necessary for improving care, but seldom done at all.

Both aspects are in fact necessary if health care is to improve. Science is needed to create and validate important, sound outcomes and cost measures, as Porter defines them, to develop a big picture of health care value and to guide policies that encourage meaningful measurement within local systems of care. We also suggest that these efforts should include defining <u>practical</u> process and outcome measures that practices and systems can begin using as stepping-stones to measuring value more comprehensively. Providers must also measure to define and solve problems in the granular delivery of care – to begin creating effective and efficient processes that are obviously lacking.

> "Practical" is underlined above because those who invent and study measures must recognize that those who use them must be able to do so without compromising their attention to patient care, a recipe for reducing value. "Quality" programs being imposed by insurers are doing just this in many cases. These self-serving cost-reducing schemes need to be set aside in favor of more uniform national policies, as the Institute of Medicine suggested 5 years ago in "Performance Measurement" [1].

We support developing value measures for research and health policy, but we will focus here on implementing practice-based measurement as critical to improving chronic disease care. We are also convinced that if providers do not lead in measuring and documenting their performance, then others will continue to do so to the disadvantage of providers and patients. Our purpose is to help load the provider train and get it moving down the tracks.

Developing a Broader "Culture of Measurement"

Why is it that physicians do not generally measure in our practices and clinical systems? It goes back to our training. While medical school faculties espouse measurement for research, and trainees are taught to value it for this purpose, measurement is seldom encouraged or taught for managing our clinical processes and outcomes. Physicians in both academia and community practices have a blind spot toward measuring our clinical performance. We will expand on the reasons for this in Chap. 24.

The continuous improvement methods that Dr. Newman described in Chap. 7 known collectively as the sciences of systems are ideal for this purpose. Like research, they depend on measurement. W. Edwards Deming first defined the knowledge required for improvement work into four domains [1, 5].

1. Knowledge of systems, such as understanding nonlinear dynamics, reliability sciences, safety sciences, and communications theory
2. Knowledge of variation, such as the ability to interpret streams of data reliably and to separate random fluctuations from meaningful ones
3. Knowledge of psychology, including understanding conflict resolution and negotiation, group process, human motivation, and creativity
4. Epistemology, especially understanding how to gain knowledge in complex environments and navigate messy real world processes

Dr. Donald Berwick has advocated for broadening the science of improvement to include both traditional science and quality improvement, each used for their best purposes [6]. Current professional and accrediting bodies including the American Association of Medical Colleges, Accrediting Committee for Graduate Medical

Education, and the Joint Commission for Accreditation of Hospitals have broadened their required competencies over the last 10 years to include these quality improvement skills. If I had known then what I do now, my 1970s Clinical Logic and Processes course would have included a heavy dose of continuous improvement methodology.

Performance measures have been used in clinical environments most commonly by the exceptional, high-performing health systems to achieve their documented successes and to differentiate themselves from other systems. A decade ago, for example, the Virginia Mason Clinic flew its administrative and clinical leadership to the Toyota Institute in Japan to learn quality improvement methods from the experts. These have also been used intuitively at first, and then studied more formally by individual physicians within clinical practices who began by asking, "How are we doing?," and then recognized that "You can't manage what you don't measure."

In fact, the scientific method and quality improvement methods both use statistical tools, but the former applies these within structured research protocols, while the latter uses them to understand what's going on in complex "real world" clinical environments and to make what's going on better. Our chapter authors are all "measurers," who have depended on measuring processes and outcomes to test and validate alternative approaches. These are often reported as before–after studies of process or outcome changes, or with serial measures derived from multiple cycles of testing, often small and rapid. We editors have purposefully sought the examples in Section IV from integrated health systems, community hospitals, and single specialty practices to debunk the notion that measuring is only possible in the big systems.

How Should You Start Measuring?

Dr. Newman has already discussed clinical process improvement methods in Chap. 7. I will focus here on using them to begin measuring and improving disease activity status for the practice's patients, the central outcome of chronic disease care.

The first rule of measuring and improving clinical performance in practices and health systems is to START. The second is to START SMALL and SIMPLE. Many well-intended improvement projects founder because they try to accomplish too much at the outset, or they test a solution before understanding the problem. Such efforts disrupt existing workflows, they are abandoned, and the status quo becomes more deeply engrained. At the beginning, those involved must get used to working in teams and must learn enough methodology to get started. Teams must get used to thinking and working in a continuous improvement mode, testing in multiple small steps. Endless planning and striving for global consensus around comprehensive solutions are the enemies of improvement. The nonadopters will beat you every time. So start, and start small and simple.

Quality improvement is supported by information technology, but at the practice level this can be as simple as an Excel spreadsheet with secure back-up and security. For example, a practice can create a list of its patients with a given chronic disease, allowing providers to say with confidence, "We have N patients with disease A, and

---

For chronic disease management, measurement begins with

- defining the disease population,
- building and maintaining a population registry,
- adopting a valid measure or measures of disease activity,
- documenting the status of each patient in the population,
- considering treatment acceleration for those with uncontrolled disease,
- and defining a standard interval for follow up measurement.

(See Example 1 in Chapter 8)

Fig. 10.2 Measurement in chronic disease

these are who they are." The population can usually be found in the ICD-9 designations within billing software systems, but it must be refined and updated, because diagnostic coding during office visits contains lots of noise. Then by applying a standardized measure of disease activity, the practice can say, "This percent of our population has active or controlled disease, and these are the ones in each group." The disease activity measure is updated for each patient at each visit, and the visit dates can be sorted to identify overdue patients. Most physicians do not currently have this information. They go from room to room and day to day, dealing with each patient at each visit as a one-off.

This report then allows the practice or health system to focus on those patients who need their time most, while setting up reliable, less resource intensive reassessment processes for the others. The time and resources to do improvement are thus rescued from the burden of low value work, and as patients' disease activity is improved, fewer of the population require more frequent and intensive care.

If data and measures are standardized, physicians often don't need to collect the required information themselves, do the disease activity calculations, or spend as much time documenting clinical data. Their time becomes dedicated to problem solving rather than finding out what's going on. Why does a patient need a physician office visit for a blood pressure check or to get a hemoglobin A1c, other than this being the simplest work to generate fee-for-service revenue?

The experience derived from this first step will generally reflect opportunities for improvement and stimulate broader improvement activities, but that's our purpose, isn't it? Once we know who our patients are and what we wish to accomplish, we can begin working on how to be more efficient, to define who on our practice team will do what, and to reduce the costs of care. This is the commitment to improvement that The Trust study (Chap. 8) identified as distinguishing high-performing health systems from the rest.

We accept Michael Porter's position that disease activity measurement for the treated population is a step toward the true goal of comprehensive value measurement, and we believe that this is the best place and way to start this journey (Fig. 10.2).

What Statistical Methods Are Useful for Clinical Process Improvement Work?

Here again insisting on perfection is too often the enemy of improvement. Simple measurements made repeatedly over time using available practice, patient, and disease population data are sufficient in many cases within clinical environments. At the other extreme, one can learn to use elegant computer programs to manage, analyze, and display data derived from large, complex health systems. There is no doubt that control charts and other graphic displays are informative and may provide superior insights, even for relatively simple variables, such as the graph of access to care measures published by the Northwestern University Rheumatology Department, and shown already in Chap. 7. Many health systems and academic institutions have management and statistical consulting services to assist in developing and executing data management strategies for more complex projects. These resources are more often used currently for business than for improving delivery of care processes and disease outcomes.

The Institute for Healthcare Improvement provides resources for measuring quality in health care [7] and books such as Thomas P. Ryan's Statistical Methods for Quality Improvement provide exhaustive treatment of quality control and applied statistics for those with an interest in all things statistical [8].

What is The Long-Term Goal of Clinical Measurement?

The goal for measuring value is best defined as providing for patients' needs at the lowest cost within individual systems of care. Process improvements are viewed in this context as mileposts on an unending journey, as is moving from practical process measures to comprehensive outcome measures. Chronic diseases are often managed at present within single specialty practices, such as rheumatoid arthritis by rheumatology. This is where the quality journey often begins, because individual practices are the units of function in most U.S. health systems. The Medicare PQRI "measures bundle" for RA provides important indicators as to how many (the numerator) of the disease population (the denominator) in a practice are receiving effective care in relation to each measure. (Table 10.1) PQRI Quality Measures exist

Table 10.1 The Medicare Physicians Quality Reporting Initiative Measures bundle for rheumatoid arthritis [9]

- Tuberculosis screening within 6 months before initiating a first biological drug
- Periodic assessment of disease activity
- Functional status assessment
- Assessment and classification of disease prognosis
- Management of risks for patients on long-term glucocorticoid treatment
- Use of disease-modifying anti-rheumatic drugs in patients with active RA

for many other chronic diseases as well [9]. Once a practice begins measuring performance for one or more of these measures, new clinical processes will need to be tested to improve the numerators.

Beyond this practice and process focus, however, achieving high-value care for most chronic disease patients requires outcome and cost measurement by cooperating providers at the health system level and over the full cycle of care – Michael Porter's vision. Otherwise the duplications, missed hand-offs, and costs multiply, while other patient needs are overlooked. Specialists do chronic disease care better, primary physicians do preventive care better, and both are required to improve value for patients. Success requires all the processes we have discussed: case finding across the system, system-level disease registries, electronic data systems, program directors and nurse coordinators, consensus algorithms, physician buy-in, decisive leadership, and continuous measurement of key indicators of processes and disease outcomes. There must be system-level programs for identifying deficits in care and a consensus to address them. This is where the journey must lead if patients are to receive great health care.

References

1. Fineberg HV. In: Performance measurement: accelerating improvement (Pathways to quality health care series). Committee on Redesigning Health Insurance Performance Measures, Payment, and Performance Improvement Programs, Board on Health Care Services, Institute of Medicine of the National Academies. Washington, DC: The National Academies Press; 2006, p. XIII.
2. Porter ME. What is value in health care? N Engl J Med. 2010;363:2477–81.
3. Supplement to reference 2. Value in health care.
4. Supplement to reference 2. Measuring health outcomes > the outcomes hierarchy.
5. Berwick DM, Finkelstein JA. Preparing medical students for the continual improvement of health and health care: Abraham Flexner and the new "public interest". Acad Med. 2010; 85:S56–65.
6. Berwick DM. The science of improvement. JAMA. 2008;299:1182–4.
7. Nolan T, Resar R, Haraden C, Griffin FA. Improving the reliability of health care. IHI Innovation Series white paper. Boston: Institute for Healthcare Improvement; 2004. www.IHI.org. Accessed 16 April 2011.
8. Ryan TP. Statistical methods for quality improvement. New York, NY: Wiley; 2000.
9. PQRI Overview. Available at: HTTP//www.cms.hhs.gov/PQRI/.

Chapter 11
Teaming: Everyone Has a Role to Play

Eric D. Newman

Keywords Teaming • Group • Belbin • Type of team • Service • Support staff
• Ownership • Leadership

The Daisy Pickers

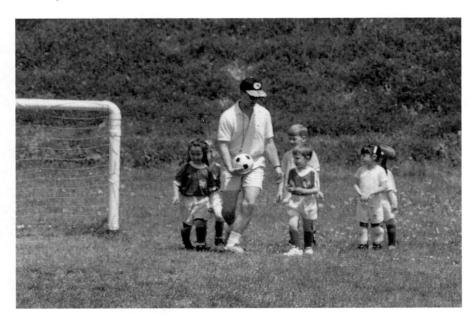

E.D. Newman, MD (✉)
Department of Rheumatology, Clinical Innovations, Division of Medicine,
Geisinger Health System, Danville, PA, USA
e-mail: arthman@aol.com

J.T. Harrington and E.D. Newman (eds.), *Great Health Care: Making It Happen*,
DOI 10.1007/978-1-4614-1198-7_11, © Springer Science+Business Media, LLC 2012

In many parts of our country, the main sport of childhood is football. I am referring of course to THE game of football – soccer. It begins at age 4 or 5. And it begins with the daisy pickers.

Soccer was my daughter's first organized gaming experience. Alyssa was 4 years old. Her first soccer game looked eerily similar to the very last game of the season. The youngsters were placed on the field like chess pieces – each with his/her specific position, and each with her/his shared skill set. I refer of course to daisy picking. And the occasional nose.

The whistle would blow, the ball would be dropped, the parents would yell, dogs and cats would dance in the streets, but very little happened on the field. Then slowly, very slowly, movement occurred. Alyssa would move her toe in a slow clockwise motion, then counterclockwise, then kick the dirt. One of her friends would bend over and snap off a dandelion. Another tyke would push the ball, kick the dirt, then pick up some grass (obviously a more advanced multitasking 4 year old). Pretty soon the field was a cacophonic chorus of disorganized little cherubs each doing their own little thing, having nothing to do with soccer. It could be deemed "the anti-team", or "humanoids in Brownian motion". Regardless, it is highly reminiscent of dysfunctional teaming – everyone does his or her own thing without an organized approach to a common goal.

After a few years, things changed. At the whistle start, the toe-sweeping daisy-pulling chorus began its 1st few measures. But one little instrument who actually understood the rules would grab the ball (sometimes with his feet, sometimes with his hands), weave in and out of the daisy pickers like a slaloming downhill skier, and bring the ball (and sometimes himself) inside the goal. The team had a shared vision, but one member was doing all the work.

Over the next few years, Alyssa's soccer team showed some degree of evolution. A few of them understood that by passing the ball and working in a cooperative fashion, they could cover more distance in less time and be more successful. Finally, around age 10, real teamwork was born. Players knew their positions, they followed the rules of engagement, and it was organized rather than disorganized mayhem. It looked like a cohesive group working together as a team, if it weren't of course for the darn parents.

So youth soccer serves as a nice metaphor for the evolution of teams and the problems they encounter. And while there is nothing finer than working with a well-oiled team, I always remember that it all started with my daisy picker.

Eric D. Newman.

We'll begin this chapter with the usual didactic approach – definitions, theories, and other necessary evils to ground us in a common framework – and then we will move to the practical. Pomp then Circumstance.

Pomp

A team can be defined as a collection of people who share a common purpose (analogous to a system – a set of interdependent variables that seek to achieve a common goal). However, a team is different than a group. A group is simply a collection – such as a group of cephalopods, or a group of wombats. A team is a group where the members bring to the table complementary skills. This allows the team to balance strengths and weaknesses among the members and to create synergism in achieving that common goal.

Since a team has many members, there must be an optimal team size. It is, of course, 4. Well, 3.7 really, but I rounded up. For those of you with a greater interest in the science of teaming, I refer you to the many works of Dr. Meredith Belbin [1].

Table 11.1 Belbin's nine roles within effective teams

Role	Description
Plant	The creative team member who helps solve the difficult problems
Resource Investigator	The one who can effectively network – bring resources together
Chairman/Coordinator	The member who assures parity among the members and seeks everyone's input
Shaper	The driven member who enjoys a challenge and for whom pressure is not a problem
Monitor-evaluator	The analytic member who views all options and seeks to place the team on the correct path
Team worker	The member who focuses on the interrelationships between members to assure a positive experience
Company worker/implementer	The practical member who can redesign systems to produce the needed results
Completer finisher	The team member who has a keen eye for details, is meticulous in their approach, and keeps track of the project timeline
Specialist	The member who brings their unique specialty knowledge to the group

Dr. Belbin, a British theorist and researcher, performed seminal work in the area of teams and teaming in the 1970s.

Dr. Belbin's 1981 book, *Management Teams*, summarized this work. He postulated that for a team to be effective, it needed to have members who could fulfill a number of key roles. He originally defined eight key roles, but a ninth – the specialist role – was added later (Table 11.1). The same person could naturally fulfill several roles, as they often cluster behaviorally within individuals. Other roles are less compatible and would likely reside within different team members. Of note is that to fulfill these nine roles, a team does not need to have nine members – in fact, according to Dr. Belbin, the optimal team number is 4. As you review the roles in Table 11.1, reflect back on the various teams of which you have been a member – the successful and unsuccessful ones. What roles did you typically play? What roles did you see in others? The roles in Table 11.1 should have face validity for you in terms of being important characteristics of well-working teams – you look at the nine factors and think "oh yeah, that's right, that's who should be in our team."

In addition to the key roles that members play within a team, the team itself may be characterized into different types [2]. Teams can be dependent or independent in their organization. *A dependent team* is one where success can only be met if the team members cooperate. In this type of team, the members may specialize into performing different tasks. A successful healthcare team could be such an example – each member plays a different role, but successful healthcare delivery cannot be achieved just by a nurse or by a physician in isolation. *An independent team* is one where each member performs similar functions, and the performance of one team member in general does not affect the success of another team member. A healthcare example could be a team of patient liaisons – each similarly skilled, doing similar tasks, with independent successes or failures.

Another type of team is *the self-managed team.* In this team scenario, the team leader does not function with a position of authority. Instead of providing the direction and giving orders, the leader delegates the decision-making to the team itself, usually by consensus. Self-managed teams are often tasked with developing and operational-izing complex projects that span different areas across a system. Many of the projects you will read about in Part IV, have some elements of a self-managed team.

A *project team* is a team that is formed to serve a discrete and self-limited pur-pose. The team members may originate from disparate parts of an organization, but they are brought together in this venue to solve a specific problem or develop a specific program. Another team derivative, commonly in healthcare, is the multidis-ciplinary team. In this type of team, specialists dealing with different aspects of the same problem come together to provide a unique, robust, and comprehensive care experience. An example might be the development of a wound care team, which could involve team members from vascular surgery, dermatology, plastic surgery, nutrition, etc.

The final team type is *the virtual team.* Virtual teams are a by-product of our electronic culture. Virtual team members work in an interdependent fashion across different organizations, across geography, and across time. By their nature, the vir-tual team members may be diverse not only by skills, but by cultural characteristics as well – be they from different counties, countries, or continents. Given that in 2001, an estimated 19 million Americans worked from a location other than a tradi-tional workplace, it is likely you have already experienced working on a team where one or more members were present on a video monitor. I am waiting for a system that can project lifelike avatars in fake business locations, so the other team mem-bers cannot see that I am really on the beach in the Caribbean. Just have to figure out how they mask the sound of waves crashing. I'll get right on it.

Circumstance

Now that we are done with the formal educational session, we can move on to the IMHO section. IMHO (In my humble opinion), effective teaming can be summed up in five words: Natasha, Teresa, Bernie, Kim, and Bonnie. The names have not been changed, because there is no need to protect the innocent. They are guilty as charged.

These five ladies form our rheumatology nursing team. They are an extraordi-nary group. Each is cut from a completely different mold, yet each contributes in a way that the value gained is larger than the sum of the parts. $1 + 1 + 1 + 1 + 1 = 27$, at least. And that's if one of them is on lunch break.

Our nursing team is one of several teaming units. We have a front desk team, an office assistant team, a physician team, a trainee (fellow) team, a clinical nurse spe-cialist team, a DXA team, a scheduling services team, and an operations manager team. Well, technically we only have a single operations manager, but she does the work of two people, so I thought I would call her a team. Together, we form the Department of Rheumatology team.

So what's so special about our team? Let me share some insights about our team's philosophy, structure, mode of functioning, and how we interact. But first, let me share an anecdote. We recently had an unannounced visit from an unnamed regulatory body. They came to check on our functioning and compliance with a myriad of health regulatory codes and statutes. This in-depth evaluation included observing our processes and firing away questions at our Rheumatology team members.

At the end of the review, the lead person came up to me and said, "Dr. Newman, your team passed with flying colors, but we do have an observation and question for you." Having just returned from lunch, I awaited with baited breath. She continued, "As we interviewed the members of your team, we found them to be .... unusually .... happy. Can you explain this?" As if *happy in healthcare* was an oxymoron! I hesitated for a moment, then pensively replied, "Yes, ... yes I can. You see that small vent. No not that one, the smaller one in the corner? That's where we pump in the nitrous oxide. It keeps 'em smiling."

Apparently, and I did not know this, some regulatory reviewers are missing a section of the dorsal pons responsible for the coordinated production of laughter. I guess they were looking for something more profound than an empty, gaseous reply. The truth is their happiness does not come from being nice to them, or even paying them better. It's about satisfaction in their job. It's about a sense of worth, and a simple, shared, common purpose. I refer of course to improving the care of those we serve – our patients.

Healthcare is a service industry. In fact, I think it's one of the most important service industries. What could be fundamentally more important than service to improve the quality of health for our fellow human beings? So to that end, about 10 years ago, our department began a journey of self-discovery and restructuring. Our trigger was participating in the Institute for Healthcare Improvement's IDCOP program. IDCOP stood for Idealized Design of the Clinical Office Practice, and our focus was to improve the access to care for patients with rheumatic diseases [3].

We recognized early on that if we were to be successful, we needed to think differently about our team. We lived in the typical world where the job of the scheduler and office assistant was to play block and tackle for (i.e., "protect") the physician. This system was feudalistic and hierarchical. The physician was at the top of the food chain. The physicians were called "staff physicians." Everyone else was called "support staff." We told them their station in life by what we called them.

We recognized that if really wanted to improve access, that model had to be replaced by one where the patient was the center of our universe, and where all of our "support staff" played an equally important role in delivering optimal care. This type of Musketeer philosophy (one-for-all and all-for-one) took several years – first to get buy-in, and then to get ownership. It required all of us to think differently. Physicians needed to be there when their patients needed them and do today's work today. In addition, they needed to move away from making judgments about patients based on their own personal value scale by trying to see how it looked from a patient's perspective.

An excellent example of this was physician cancelations. Not a big deal, right? "I only canceled two patients for next week." But what of those two patients? One was in significant pain and fear and had waited a month to be seen. The other patient's daughter had taken off of work to transport her mom to the clinic. This last minute decision significantly and adversely affected the lives of those who we purportedly were trying to help. Think systems – we need to consider the upstream and downstream effect of every decision we make.

In addition to moving our physicians to a more patient-centric philosophy, the other challenge was getting our costaff (no longer called "support staff") to feel comfortable making decisions, speaking up at meetings, etc. It took many months, but by empowering them to do so, rewarding them verbally when they did, being consistent, and articulating a shared philosophy of "you get it – you own it," we have achieved a team structure and philosophy that allows us to be more successful and more content in our jobs.

What about leadership structure for our teams? At our healthcare system, we pair a physician leader with an administrative leader at virtually all levels. At the department level, a physician director is paired with an operations manager. These two individuals work synergistically to lead their local team's system of care. In most cases, these two individuals consider themselves equals, as opposed to the administrative partner assisting the physician leader. The teams where this relationship holds (equal partners) are the strongest teams.

So the path I am advocating for you is to consider redesigning your current team structure and philosophy, so your team gets up in the morning thinking about how they can best care for the patients in need. This brings me to the final issue of hiring new team members – and two mistakes I have made that I want you to avoid.

The first mistake is the belief that simply introducing a new hire into your new environment is sufficient for that person to adapt and adopt with time. Even if it's crystal clear what the philosophy and practice style is, the new hire will need help – education and repeated feedback – to break old habits and form better ones. I have found that new physicians need more of that help than new costaff – perhaps because as an ilk we tend to be free thinkers, and fitting into a mold where we are not top dog is anathema.

The second mistake is the belief that we can actually interview someone and predict his or her ability to adjust, adapt, and most importantly thrive, simply by the usual interview process. I have had physicians with excellent pedigrees and fantastic recommendations who simply could not fit into our style. I have had costaff who were either unknowns, or simply had little training, who have become the pillars of support for our team. It's easy to get fooled. One of my favorite quotes along this line is from Gilbert and Sullivan's The H.M.S. Pinafore: "Things are seldom what they seem, skin milk masquerades as cream."

To avoid making the wrong decision, I would advocate whenever possible that you consider a several month trial period to make sure that you have hired the right person. In addition, it's better to hire someone who appears to truly share your belief system, but you need to heavily train, than to hire someone pre-trained when you question their ability to adapt and adopt. Nonadoptors are the killers of quality improvement – avoid them at all costs.

So we have discussed that successful teaming in healthcare is about the right people, the right infrastructure, and the right mantra. I think the Cleveland Clinic says it best with their sound-bite approach, displayed about every 3 ft.– "Patients First." Go Team.

References

1. Belbin M. Management teams. London: Heineman; 1981.
2. http://en.wikipedia.org/wiki/Team.
3. Newman ED, Harrington TH, Olenginski TP, Perruquet JL, McKinley K. "The rheumatologist can see you now": successful implementation of an advanced access model in a rheumatology practice. Arthritis Care and Research. 2004;51:253–7.

Chapter 12
How Providers Should Be Paid

Eric D. Newman

Keywords Value • RVUs • Payment systems • Accountable care organizations • Global payments • Bundled payments • Prometheus payments • Compensation plan

"Something for Nothing and Nothing for Something"

What we want (whether we realize it or not) is to be paid fairly for delivering services of high value. At it is simplest, value can be considered as a ratio – with quality and efficiency in the numerator and cost in the denominator. As such, improving quality and efficiency while simultaneously reducing cost helps to create better value. Let me share two personal anecdotes describing the extremes of the value formula — something for nothing and nothing for something.

My son Nathaniel and daughter Alyssa (now 23 and 21) grew up with an unusual relationship – as best buddies. Both had strong musical backgrounds. In their high school years, for a brief period they combined their talents as a brother–sister act – Alyssa on vocals, and Nathaniel on guitar. Their first performance was at a cafe in our town (Fig. 12.1). They brought their own equipment and set themselves up. They were fabulous – song after song, filled with sweet passion and high energy. They performed to a sell-out crowd. Now let us examine their value formula. They delivered exceptional quality, they did so efficiently, they cost next to nothing (both received 1 free nonalcoholic drink) – their value was almost infinite. But they received no compensation. Something for nothing.

Switch gears to my childhood. Every year, my parents would drive my sister and me into New York City to experience the Feast of San Gennaro Festival in the Little Italy section of Manhattan. Every year I would watch the vendor who had set up a game of chance, where the object was to toss a nickel from a distance and have it land on a plate suspended in the air. The prize was a beautiful parrot, sitting in a cage of gold. After thousands of tosses, and many years of observation, a winner finally emerged. The vendor loudly announced the event, then proceeded to grab the parrot from the gilded cage, shoved the bird into a crumpled paper bag, and handed it to the successful nickel-tosser. The man was aghast. "Whhhat about the cage'?, he stammered. The vendor leaned forward, and with a soft voice he replied in a heavy Italian accent "the cage, ahh, that's a-five hundred dollars".

E.D. Newman, MD (✉)
Department of Rheumatology, Clinical Innovations, Division of Medicine,
Geisinger Health System, Danville, PA, USA
e-mail: arthman@aol.com

J.T. Harrington and E.D. Newman (eds.), *Great Health Care: Making It Happen*,
DOI 10.1007/978-1-4614-1198-7_12, © Springer Science+Business Media, LLC 2012

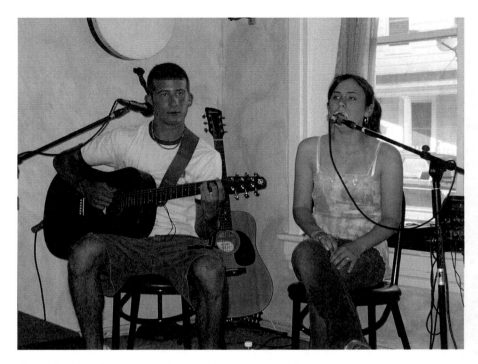

Fig. 12.1 Delivering exceptional value high quality at a minimal cost

> *The winner returned the parrot, paper bag and all. Nothing for something.*
> *We need to seek a middle ground. Improve quality of care delivery. Do so efficiently. Be*
> *mindful of costs. Get paid accordingly. Something for something. Sounds simple. Seems*
> *impossible. Let us begin*
>
> Eric D. Newman.

Physicians are paid incorrectly. We are paid more for doing more things, not for delivering better value. The old system of payment was closer to value-based reimbursement. In the old days, a physician performed certain services for a patient, and the patient paid what they thought the services were worth. This payment was based on the value delivered combined with patient's ability to pay. Gold coins for some, chickens for others, a hearty thanks for a few. But at the end of a day … it was a good day. Now we have a measurement system based on a biased indicator – RVUs (ridiculous value units), a fee for service payment system designed to drive up cost, and young physicians with untenable debts who are forced to make career decisions based on financial survivorship rather than a true calling. Moreover, it kills cooperation and paralyzes necessary change. It involves flawed measurement, incorrect incentive, and bad decision making. It is the Trifecta of Imperfecta.

We could spend (days, weeks, years, and careers) speaking about what is wrong, and we did enough of this already in Chap. 3. Instead, let us focus on some of the proposed solutions to physician payment that are out there, and begin to flesh out a model that may make some sense to you, depending on your willingness to think outside of your usual box, and the amount of mind altering substances you may have ingested before reading this chapter. We will then propose what seems like a reasonable first step toward a compensation plan in today's mixed-up reimbursement world, and finish with some principles behind how a truly novel payment system might look.

There are two pieces to this: how insurers (payers) – commercial companies, Medicare, others – pay for services provided to their clients, and how medical practices divide up these revenues among their physicians. Both pieces strongly influence what care is delivered, how, and at what cost. In most cases, if insurers pay for fragments of care with no relation to value, physicians get paid for the same. And when insurers have tried to pay differently, medical practices still pay their physicians for fragments of care based on RVUs.

Proposed Payment Systems

There are basically four physician payment experiments currently in play among insurers as alternatives to paying individual physicians and other providers fee-for-service. These include Accountable Care Organizations (ACOs), Global Payments, Bundled Payments, and Prometheus [1–4]. Each has interesting and compelling reasons why it may move us forward, but each has significant limitations, none is the magic bullet – and unfortunately none involves chickens.

Accountable Care Organizations

An ACO is a group of providers that contracts with a payer to be responsible for the quality and cost of care for a population. That group could include a hospital, a collection of physicians, or a combination, but it must include primary care physicians. The population might include all the payers clients, those with a particular disease, or those requiring a specific procedure. The ACO must be prepared to manage patients across a multitude of care settings, and it must measure and report on the quality of care delivered.

There are two potential ways an ACO could receive reimbursement. The first is a risk-taking model. In this model, the ACO would be responsible for all of the costs generated on both the inpatient and outpatient sides. The profits in this model would be determined based on two factors: meeting quality goals, and reducing costs below some preset "budget." The second is a sharing savings model, which is what Medicare is supporting through the Patient Protection and Affordable Care Act [5]. The ACO is paid in a fee-for-service methodology, but if it achieves certain quality benchmarks AND spends less than a set expense benchmark per capita, Medicare splits the savings with the ACO.

Global Payments

In the Global Payment methodology, the focus is on the resources needed to manage a population, including compensation for providers. So far so good. This payment scheme could be applied to groups of any size – a solo practice, a group practice, or a larger integrated organization. Payment would be received based on services that were provided – get paid as you go. Quality data gathering and reporting is essential. An annual target is established for the population. If the expenses are under this target, then the profits are shared. In some variations, advanced estimated payments are made, with periodic withholds and reconciliation.

Bundled Payments

The Bundled Payment concept is deceptively simple – pay a single payment for an episode of each patient's care. This episode of care is defined by a "case rate." This case rate could reflect payment for a hospitalization, a hospitalization followed by the acute posthospitalization care, or a defined time interval surrounding care for a chronic disease. The payment itself would be rendered to a hospital, which would then divide it between themselves and the providers.

As an example, the Geisinger Health System has developed a product line surrounding bundled payments known as "ProvenCare." [6] In the initial ProvenCare model involving elective coronary artery bypass graft surgery (CABG), a single payment was accepted for all required care – pre-op evaluation, inpatient care (both facility and physician), postoperative care, and complications. The payment price was based on average treatment costs plus 50% of the complication costs (calculated via historical experience). In addition, ProvenCare came with a guarantee – adherence to 40 different process-of-care measures. Nonadherence directly affected a portion of the surgeon's payment. The ProvenCare portfolio has since been extended to include elective percutaneous angioplasty, total hip replacement, cataract surgery, erythropoietin use, perinatal care, and bariatric surgery.

Prometheus Payments

Prometheus is the Greek God of forethought. However, the Prometheus of which we are speaking is an acronym for "Provider payment reform for outcomes, margins, evidence, transparency, hassle reduction, excellence, understandability and sustainability." I of course prefer the other Google definition, "Program for European Traffic with Highest Efficiency and Unprecedented Safety." A mouthful either way.

But aside from the linguistic challenge, Prometheus is a promising methodology with a lot of curb appeal. The basic concept is paying physicians, practices, or others for providing efficient care and avoiding harm. It begins with establishing an "evidenced-informed case rate," or ECR. The ECR includes all services related to that episode of care, has a defined time period, and uses evidenced-based guidelines to determine what services are covered. The ECR is adjusted to account for the individual patient's severity and complexity of disease. ECRs have been created for acute myocardial infarctions, joint replacement, diabetes, asthma, congestive heart failure, and hypertension. In addition, Prometheus calls for developing a potentially avoidable complication (PAC) pool. The PAC is based on the ECR, and is paid out either as complications occur, or as a bonus to providers if the PACs are avoided. Once the PAC pool is used up for the budget year, further costs for this care are the providers' responsibility.

A physician joins the Prometheus team and agrees to provide services for a specific part of the guidelines-based care. Physicians are paid in a fee-for-service mode for services rendered, and those services are debited against the ECR. A portion of the ECR is held back, and is paid according to a provider scorecard. That scorecard is based 70% on the individual provider's measures, and 30% on the overall team's measures. This Musketeer philosophy (one for all and all for one) helps promote teamwork.

To summarize, each of these proposed alternatives has its positives, but unfortunately they also have problems related to incentives, unintended consequences, and management complexities. We can think of lots of the latter, and I will bet you can come up with your own list. We suspect, however, that payers will go right ahead implementing an array of such programs, and that provider groups will be burdened with sorting things out.

A Physician Compensation Plan for Today

We will next move from 50,000 to 5 ft to consider how practices and medical groups might best compensate their physicians to achieve high performance, in spite of how the insurers calculate revenues. We will describe a plan that is a first step toward rewarding some of the right things, and then finish with some bold thoughts about where this should and could move next. We are talking here about the incentives providers create for themselves. This last section will not be for the faint of heart.

I have worked for the past 25 years at the same institution. Over that time, I have seen 25 different compensation plans. Well, 27 really. However, willingness among our physicians has emerged recently to move beyond the typical EWYK (eat what you kill) compensation paradigm. While we are far from perfect, physicians have at least started thinking that there is more to life than RVUs.

Dr. Harrington and I have combined our collective compensation, and decompensation experiences into a physician salary + incentive approach that we believe takes a first step in the right direction. Mind you, this is not a final solution, just a way to begin thinking about moving from point A to point B. *No matter how, and how many different ways a practice is paid by insurers for providing patient care, once you move beyond solo practice, the internal allocation of expenses and compensation will reflect what the physicians' value, and will determine how they function.* We are impressed that those medical practices and systems in the U.S. and elsewhere those who pay their physicians a market-based salary are providing higher value compared to those who continue to pay for fragments.

Here is the way we see it:

Physicians' Total Compensation is market-based and is divided into base, incentive, and benefits:

Base

- Paid monthly
- Components

  - Expectation: work RVUs to specialty median benchmarks
  - Penalty: below benchmark work triggers semiannual downward adjustment of base
  - Bonus (possible): if profits exceed the budget, individuals receive a bonus

Incentive

- Paid on a less frequent basis (e.g., quarterly)
- Components (examples)

  - Practice management
  - Academics
  - Citizenship
  - Quality
  - Care coordination/integration
  - Patient satisfaction
  - Referring/receiving physician satisfaction
  - Whatever else is important to achieving practice goals, ideally defined through business planning

Benefits – Let us not forget to make physicians aware of these costs to the practice.

There are several caveats of note:

- Effective leadership is required to move compensation away from EWYK.
- Objective measures for the incentive components are required.
- Focus must be maintained. The tendency is to create a large number of incentive components, which become unmanageable for physicians and managers.
- Incentives should be paid as close to the required efforts as possible. The difficult part is that some important incentives cannot be meaningfully measured frequently.
- Consider a performance scale for the incentive components to encourage excellence and discourage complacency, not just Yes or No. e.g.,

  - Minimal (50% of incentive %)
  - Target (100% of incentive %)

– Ideal (150% of incentive %)
– Below minimal (0% of incentive %)

This approach is not perfect – no plan is – but it does weaken volume drivers, replacing them with market-based income expectations related to meeting work expectations and delivering measurable value. Incentives can be assigned to teams, not just individuals. Appropriate incentives will encourage value-producing behaviors. But the devil is always in the details, and several pitfalls must be avoided:

First, paying a bonus for "beating budget" may just lead to chasing profits instead of work volume. Second, a salary + incentive-based plan assumes that developing a realistic budget is a science. This could not be further from the truth. Budgeting for the base is predictable, but budgeting for the incentives is not, because how much is earned may vary greatly, as from 0 to 150% for any measure in our example. Budgeting a maximum amount for incentives is necessary; paying what is not distributed to those who did earn theirs' might accelerate behavior changes. Sometimes it is that the system goal is unachievable, and sometimes it is simply how the slices of pie are divided as the budget moves from system to service line to division to department. And unforeseen events can always blow up the budget, as in the monies to fund the compensation plan did not reach budget.

Third, the ability of physicians to "beat budget" to earn a productivity bonus is ripe for "gaming," because the dollars received vary for different categories of work. As examples, RVUs are weighted against primary care and cognitive subspecialists, and it is much easier to move the bar by doing procedures than it is by seeing clinic patients. The playing field must be level for incentives to be seen as transparent and equitable. Fourth, incentive payments would be most effective if other care team members – nurses, front desk, secretaries, and extenders – were similarly engaged and incentivized. Sadly, this type of co-alignment rarely happens.

Finally, it is unclear what the correct percentage of total compensation should be for the base and incentive. A significant base is required for personal income management, and a significant incentive component is necessary to reward desired behaviors. For what it is worth, compensation plans that incorporate incentives often have a base:incentive ratio of 80:20 or 70:30.

How We Should Be Paid Ideally, and for What?

Here is where I do the future vision thing, jumping from where we are to where we need to be – one impossible leap. The systems person in me cannot get away from thinking that to deliver effective chronic disease management – improve quality, be more efficient, reduce costs – we need to organize, cooperate, integrate, and iterate broadly. We need to have a set of common goals and incentives. We need to agree on each other's roles, and help each other out – primary care, specialty care, insurers, and patients all dancing cheek to cheek. In essence, remove the silos; think differently. And we need to be paid for our successes in achieving this vision, if we are to get there.

Table 12.1 Patient Centered Medical Home (PCMH)-specialty integration principles

• Use of effective communication
• Service focused
• Excellence in access
• Patient-centric care philosophy
• Multiple care delivery choices (e.g., face-to-face, telephone, email, telemedicine)
• Use electronics effectively
• Health promotion
• Integration of services
• Continuous process improvement
• Evidence-based approach
• Philosophy of measurement

Think it is impossible? The "Success Stories Told by Champions" in Part IV would argue that this is possible, and that it has already begun. Some organizations are meeting these high expectations in spite of a whole variety of different compensation plans; those whose physician compensation incentivizes these behaviors are doing best for their patients.

I am currently involved at Geisinger in a project to successfully integrate our specialty and primary care to better manage patients with chronic diseases. We have most of the right players at the table – primary care, specialty care, healthcare insurer, and our innovations team. Several pilots are underway to reexamine and redesign the delivery of care. The major limitations I have found to date are:

1. The lack of software to effectively manage populations across a continuum of care, geography, and task management needs.
2. Getting people to think of truly creative ideas, and outside their own silos.

What has been pleasantly refreshing is the excitement of the participating groups, on both the primary care side and the specialty side. We have engendered a sense of pride (we can *do this*), ownership (*we* can do this), and confidence (we *can* do this). Time will tell whether we can translate this into effective outcomes, but it will be a tremendous learning experience which can only serve us to do better.

So how should we be paid for such improvement efforts? Maybe we should think of this in terms of tools, infrastructure, integration principles, and measures. We should be "given" the tools as part of the government's overall electronic infrastructure initiative, because we cannot pay for them out-of-pocket. Then, we should be paid for creating and maintaining the infrastructure, following the integration principles, and improving the value measures – all successes based on teamwork.

Table 12.1 highlights the integration principles that these Patient Centered Medical Home (PCMH)-Specialty integration groups would espouse. Measures of success would need to be derived for these core principles and reimbursed accordingly. The integrated groups would be co-responsible for improving the entire bundle of measures. For example, the same diabetic measures may be co-owned by

PCMH and Endocrinology, regardless of who is assigned responsibility for actual direct patient management. This engages the PCMH and the specialists to work together to improve care for the population at risk and with disease.

So .... pay for developing and maintaining infrastructure, pay for objectively following the core integration principles, pay for improving co-attributable quality/efficiency/cost measures. Notice nowhere did I mention that you got paid for doing more to patients.

The widget is dead and buried. Long live the patient.

References

1. Terry KJ. Physician payment reform: what it could mean to doctors – part 1: Accountable Care Organizations. 2010. http://www.medscape.com/viewarticle/726537. Accessed 31 Oct 2010.
2. Kane L. Physician payment reform: what it could mean to doctors – part 2: Global payments. 2010. http://www.medscape.com/viewarticle/726776. Accessed 31 Oct 2010.
3. Reese SM. Physician payment reform: what it could mean to doctors – part 3: bundled payments. 2010. http://www.medscape.com/viewarticle/727115. Accessed 31 Oct 2010.
4. Terry KJ. Physician payment reform: what it could mean to doctors – part 4: Prometheus payment. 2010. http://www.medscape.com/viewarticle/727737. Accessed 31 Oct 2010.
5. Berwick DM. Launching Accountable Care Organizations – the proposed rule for the Medicare shared savings program. New Engl J Med. 2011;364:e32.
6. Casale AS, Paulus RA, Selna MJ, et al. "ProvenCareSM": a provider-driven pay-for-performance program for acute episodic cardiac surgical care. Ann Surg. 2007;246(4):613–23.

Part IV
Success Stories Told by Champions: Boldly Going Where Few Have Gone Before

J. Timothy Harrington

> *They are all saying the same thing! (Abigail Cantor, Systems design consultant).*
>
> *In 2006, I became interested in how to keep track of osteoporosis patients over time and across our health system, and then for those patients with several chronic diseases that were managed by multiple specialties. It is these latter patients who present the greatest challenges and fall through the cracks most frequently. I asked my industrial engineering colleague, Abigail Cantor, to interview specialists in diabetes, congestive heart failure, hypertension, rheumatoid arthritis, chronic kidney disease, and osteoporosis in order to understand their management processes and how these might be better coordinated. They each regaled Abigail with their highly personalized care of their favorite disease. When the interviews were over, Abigail declared, "They are all saying the same thing," and she drew up a single chronic disease management algorithm that provides a vision for standardizing and coordinating clinical work across disease populations and specialties (Fig. IV.1).*
>
> *J. Timothy Harrington*

This part is the centerpiece of our book. Each chapter author or team describes the program they have developed and sustained that provides great health care for an important chronic disease, or in the case of the final chapter by Dr. Martha Twaddle, for end of life care. These programs are widely recognized within their own specialties. The authors are the doers. The details of treatments and the specific challenges may differ by disease; the communities and health systems may differ; but the common threads of personal inspiration, the continuous improvement of

J.T. Harrington, MD
Division of Rheumatology, University of Wisconsin School of Medicine and Public Health, Madison, WI, USA

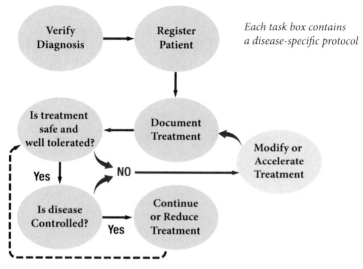

Disease Monitoring Cycle:
Frequency is based on disease and treatment monitoring protocols

Fig. IV.1 Chronic disease management algorithm

care, and the disease management principles that emerge from these success stories are similar. The editors will comment briefly at the end of each chapter to highlight the relationships to our teachings in Parts II and III.

The enthusiastic responses to our invitations from these national experts suggested that our book idea might be on the right track. Finding them was itself a unique experience. A few we knew personally or by reputation. Otherwise we discovered our champions by contacting the best people we knew in each disease specialty. They suggested the person that would be their first choice. That person sometimes said, "I'll do it, but the person you really want is … " Once we got to the best of the best, they always said "Yes!"

Chapter 13
Diabetes: Everyone's Number One Priority

Richard S. Beaser, Kenneth Snow, Jo-Anne M. Rizzotto, Julie Brown, and Martin J. Abrahamson

Keywords Diabetes • Joslincare • Partnership • Communication • Customer service • Multidiscipinary teams • Joslin affiliates • Joslin professional education continuum

Diabetes tops most clinicians' list of most challenging conditions to treat, largely due to the complexity and clinical fluidity of its treatment targets; the overlap of its clinical implications onto other medical conditions such as vascular, renal, ophthalmologic, and neurologic diseases; and the need to extend treatments beyond mere medication prescription into the challenging realm of patient self-management training and lifestyle changes.

Type 2 diabetes predominates compared to type 1 and is often seen in the context of an array of cardiometabolic risk factors, including hypertension, dyslipidemia, and weight management, that require complex nonpharmacologic and pharmacologic interventions. Further, the ability to deliver quality diabetes care is not dependent solely on the knowledge and skill of a clinician, but also on the clinical care systems in which he or she practices, and contributions of other clinicians with different but complementary skills. About 90% of people with diabetes are cared for by primary care providers (PCPs) [1], perhaps complemented by area specialty resources to augment what their own practice cannot provide directly. No person can decide to do a good job, and make that wish come true! For all involved, optimizing diabetes treatment and outcomes takes a coordinated team.

We are seeing epidemics of diabetes, obesity, and cardiovascular disease (CVD) [2], with CVD associated with the cause of death in approximately 65% of persons with diabetes [3]. In 2008, the Centers for Disease Control and Prevention estimated

R.S. Beaser, MD(✉) • K. Snow, MD • J.-A.M. Rizzotto, MEd, RD, LDN, CDE
• J. Brown, CCMEP • M.J. Abrahamson, MD, FACP
Joslin Diabetes Center, Harvard Medical School, Boston, MA, USA
e-mail: Richard.Beaser@joslin.harvard.edu

J.T. Harrington and E.D. Newman (eds.), *Great Health Care: Making It Happen*,
DOI 10.1007/978-1-4614-1198-7_13, © Springer Science+Business Media, LLC 2012

the prevalence of diabetes in the U.S. at 7.8% of the total population, or 23.6 million people, with 17.9 million diagnosed and 5.7 million undiagnosed [4], and the numbers continuing to grow [5]. Unfortunately, the care being delivered is not optimal, particularly in terms of the services offered and goals achieved in primary care settings [6, 7]. Data from the National Health and Nutrition Examination Survey (NHANES) show that only 49.8% of adults with diabetes achieved the recommended A1C target of less than 7%, and 29.7% had an A1C above 8% [8]. Shortfalls due to the failure of clinicians to initiate or intensify therapy when indicated, referred to as clinical inertia, are a significant healthcare delivery concern [9].

Specialty diabetes practices are designed to address many of the clinical care and practice system obstacles to optimized care, but can impact only a fraction of people with diabetes. To improve diabetes care nationally, we have to use leading diabetes specialty care settings as models of care, and explore how their expertise can be leveraged to help regional specialty centers and local primary care practices provide more comprehensive diabetes management services. To this end, many groups have attempted to codify diabetes care through the development and promulgation of clinical guidelines to help clinicians determine the course of treatment. Guideline use would provide a common care template, theoretically easing communication and providing indications for therapies and consultative care assistance. They could also help clinicians self-define what services a primary vs. specialty practice might provide and determine clear indications for consultative referrals. However, data from a recent Joslin Diabetes Center needs assessment survey to determine the focus of continuing medical education (CME) efforts indicated that PCPs are not following national guidelines for initiation and advancement of treatment for patients with type 2 diabetes, identifying patients at increased cardiometabolic risk, or reporting confidence in treating patients, particularly with insulin [10].

The clinical inertia typical of current care, with its less aggressive therapeutic advancement and failure to achieve goals or utilize evidence-based guidelines as roadmaps for coordinated care, has resulted in diabetes treatments not reaching full potential. To address this concern, we put forth the Joslin model: the core diabetes specialty center in Boston, the affiliated specialty centers throughout the United States, and the efforts of the Professional Education department to provide knowledge and practice systems support to PCPs to help them work more effectively in their own communities for the betterment of the millions of people who have diabetes.

The Care Model at the Joslin Diabetes Center, Boston: "JoslinCare"

The Joslin Diabetes Center in Boston, Massachusetts, founded by Dr. Elliott P. Joslin in 1898, is recognized as a world-class comprehensive, multidisciplinary outpatient education and care facility for people with diabetes (Joslin Clinic), and a leading diabetes research center ranking in the top five percent of all research centers in grant support from the National Institutes of Health. Joslin Diabetes Center is also recognized for its outreach programs, which include professional education and its affiliated centers network. The process of coordinated team care by diabetes-focused endocrinologists, nurse practitioners, diabetes educators, and patients working in concert to manage this condition and its related complications has become known as "JoslinCare." Joslin Clinic provides care for more than 20,000 patients drawn mostly from the Boston metropolitan area.

JoslinCare is a philosophy and systems approach to care of the person with diabetes that features care provided by teams of providers based on three key elements: partnership, communication, and customer service. Each of four multidisciplinary teams in the Adult diabetes section provides general diabetes care but also focuses on a particular cohort of patients: pregnant or elderly patients, ethnic-specific patients, patients with eating disorders or obesity, and patients using insulin pumps and sensors. A separate pediatric section provides team-based care for children and adolescents with diabetes.

Each adult team includes dedicated endocrinologists/diabetologists, nurse educators, a nurse practitioner, a medical assistant, dietitians, an exercise physiologist, and a care coordinator. All of the nonphysician caregivers on JoslinCare teams are Certified Diabetes Educators with advanced training. Teams share the services of ophthalmologists trained in retinal disease, mental health professionals, nephrologists, an onsite laboratory, and the Joslin Vision Network retinal screening resources. These practice groups meet bimonthly to review clinical cases, protocols of care, operational issues, and clinical and operational metrics of performance. Administrative staff coordinates all the scheduling and administrative support from a shared clinical administrative unit and patient information is maintained in the electronic health record. All follow-up communication and clinic appointments for patients are directed to or scheduled with team members.

Strategic Goals for JoslinCare

The goals of the JoslinCare construct are to provide a platform to integrate the clinic sections, develop a sound educational curriculum, and increase staff awareness of the importance of their role in the care model. Its structure is embedded in the electronic systems utilized. We strive to make JoslinCare consistent with the chronic care model and to ensure that the system of care meets the educational, medical, and psychological needs of patients by providing modern, evidence-based, coordinated care. This approach should meet the individual needs of the patient and ensure improved self-management and empowerment. The system should facilitate adherence to care, follow specialty referral guidelines, maximize efficiency, and improve access to care. It should meet or exceed pay-for-performance and other benchmark expectations. The JoslinCare model is utilized by healthcare systems locally, nationally, and internationally through the Affiliate programs, and is the template upon which much of our professional education is based.

Initial Visit (Fig. 13.1 JoslinCare Initial Visit)

At their initial visit, patients meet with the team care coordinator who checks vital signs, does initial laboraroty work, and lists the patient's medications. A non-mydriatic (undilated) digital image of the fundi (JVN) is taken next, after which the patient sees the endocrinologist/diabetologist and then a diabetes educator (JoslinCare Partner), who together develop a clinical and behavioral management plan with the patient. Patients are expected to participate actively in determining treatment and setting therapy and behavior change goals, including frequency of blood glucose monitoring; lifestyle changes for nutrition and exercise; and blood pressure, A1C, and lipid targets. The plan may include referrals to nephrologists, psychologists, or ophthalmologists within Joslin, or to external cardiologists, podiatrists, or other specialists. It may also include key care instructions and plans for follow-up laboratories, diagnostic tests, and education.

Success and Challenges

Joslin has been measuring clinical outcomes since the implementation of the JoslinCare model and electronic medical record. Our preliminary data suggest that compared to patients cared for by external providers, those who receive regular care at Joslin over many years have lower rates of end-stage kidney disease (Joslin 7.7%, external 14%) and early-stage retinopathy (Joslin 22.2%, external 27.3%). Similarly, 57% of patients seen for 10–15 years have early-stage retinopathy compared to 86% in the Wisconsin Study [11]. The data also suggest that patients treated at Joslin for 15 years or more have lower complication rates than those who receive care for shorter periods. Joslin patients who receive nephrology and ophthalmology services in addition to education and clinical care in adult diabetes have a greater reduction in A1C 1 year after their initial appointment compared to those patients who only see the diabetologist and diabetes educator (0.83% reduction compared to 0.37%).

JoslinCare New Patient Flow

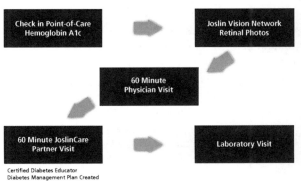

Fig. 13.1 Unique multidisciplinary approach to diabetes management

The additional cost of Joslin's multidisciplinary team and expanded role for educators vs. a standard, non-team approach was estimated at $340 per year. The savings in treatment for complications due to JoslinCare were estimated to be $250 per patient per year with type 1 diabetes. This estimate is based on Joslin's average A1C reduction of 1.2% for our patients in the first year of care, coupled with data on costs and incidence of complications reported by the American Diabetes Association [12]. A similar analysis for Joslin's patients with type 2 diabetes suggested a cost savings of $450 per patient. Reductions in blood pressure from Joslin teams' more intensive management showed even greater cost savings, in the range of $1,400 per year per patient with type 2 diabetes.

Ongoing Care

The frequency of follow-up of patients depends on the type of diabetes, complexity of therapy, and the type and extent of education classes or programs prescribed for the patient. Follow-up plans may include one-on-one appointments with nurse educators, dietitians, and exercise physiologists; participation in weight management, intensive diabetes management, and education programs; and training and initiation of insulin pump and glucose sensor use. Medical follow-up is provided by physicians or nurse practitioners who specialize in diabetes management. Joslin attempts wherever possible to participate in a collaborative care model with patients' PCPs; we believe that this communication with PCPs is essential.

Medical management of diabetes includes counseling and treatment of all cardiovascular risk factors, and Joslin endocrinologists often prescribe medications and lifestyle modifications to address a patient's high blood pressure, elevated cholesterol, or routine coronary concerns. Patients needing more specialized cardiology, vascular, or podiatry care, or procedures related to these subspecialties, are referred to appropriate specialists at nearby Beth Israel Deaconess Medical Center (BIDMC). For pregnant patients with preexisting or gestational diabetes, Joslin coordinates care with obstetric clinicians at BIDMC.

Looking Ahead

Joslin is proud of our care model but continually aspires to improve that model and the health outcomes for our patients. Recognizing the success of the coordinated care model, Joslin seeks to expand the range of coordinated care to include expanded "priority" testing and easier access to specialty care, where appropriate, to prevent or slow the progression of complications. As we look to the future, we expect our model of care to leverage technology to facilitate education and management of diabetes by using patient portals and other electronic systems to enable patients to access Joslin educational and medical management tools and to enhance communication between patients and all their care providers.

Diabetes Care in the Community:
The Joslin Model for Specialty Outreach

In the context of the epidemic of diabetes, obesity, and the cardiometabolic syndrome, an important healthcare delivery question is how to move optimized treatment beyond the specialty centers into the realm of the PCPs. Centers of excellence in diabetes satisfy many needs in our current healthcare system, but cannot provide total care for the approximately 8% of the population who have diabetes, much less the estimated growth of 1.5 million new cases annually [4]. The demonstrated relationship between improved diabetes control and decreased rates of complications [13–15] makes the ability to extend optimized care extremely important for both health and economic reasons.

Concurrently, multiple new therapies and technological advances are becoming available. In the past two decades we have seen eight new classes of noninsulin therapies, several new synthetic insulins, the move beyond vial and syringe to convenient insulin pens and pumps, and more sophisticated monitoring devices including continuous glucose monitors that can reveal full-day glycemic patterns. While these advancements provide multiple options to better control diabetes, they have made the approach to care more complex and require greater expertise among physicians to benefit patients.

While primary care physicians can still treat the majority of people with diabetes, recognition of the benefit of aggressive diabetes management as well as the range of treatment options to reduce cardiometabolic risk can present an overwhelming burden to many of these clinicians. More importantly than ever before, the presence of centers of excellence in diabetes provides primary care physicians and their patients' access to the highest level of diabetes care available for that subset for whom this level of care is needed. Yet the question remains, how to make the expertise of these centers available to the broad reach of PCPs and their patients, and to systematize interactions between these two segments to improve both quality and quantity of care.

Not all endocrinologists are "diabetologists" with a specialty focus on diabetes in either their interests or the comprehensiveness of their practice systems. While they likely have diabetes expertise, Joslin believes that the focus on comprehensive diabetes centers of excellence has become important. In recognition of this need for more diabetes-focused centers of excellence outside of our center in Boston and comparable university diabetes programs throughout the country, Joslin Diabetes Center created our affiliated program model. Joslin Affiliates serve as centers of excellence for patients needing referral, coordinating care among multiple specialty providers, and offering regional resources for professional and patient education support and materials. This model connects the Boston center and our mission of excellence in diabetes care with like-minded institutions elsewhere around the country. Modeled after Joslin Clinic, Joslin Affiliates utilize the same team approach to care and leverage similar regional specialty services to complete the needed spectrum of care that we believe should be available through a diabetes center of excellence.

Joslin provides the Affiliate team with policies and procedures mimicking those at Joslin Clinic. Ongoing interaction between Joslin and each Affiliate throughout the year includes on-site Affiliate visits from a Boston team consisting of a physician, educator, and administrative staff to guarantee the quality of Affiliate care. An annual meeting in Boston for Affiliate staff provides collective brainstorming sessions, knowledge updates, and opportunities to share "best practices." Ongoing conference calls and virtual meetings for all members of the team help to assure a network-wide standard of care. Finally, quality metrics for each affiliate are reviewed and compared across the Affiliate network as well as to Joslin Clinic to further assure that the quality of care is consistent with that provided in Boston.

For the foreseeable future, growing numbers of both people with diabetes and therapeutic options will increase the need for similar growth in the number of centers of excellence in diabetes as provided by Joslin-affiliated programs. Joslin needs like-minded partners who recognize the value of providing world-class diabetes care at a level beyond what would be available from primary care physicians alone, but who also look to serve as a resource for primary care physicians to assist them in treating patients who are best managed in the primary care setting. Optimizing diabetes treatment and outcomes takes a coordinated team, and that team must include the primary care network surrounding a diabetes center of excellence.

The Joslin Model in the Primary Care Setting: Performance Improvement Education

As noted, while a key facet of the Joslin approach to improving diabetes treatment nationwide is replication of the Joslin Clinic model in regional centers of excellence, the next step in that continuum is to emanate support and expertise to area primary care practices through both patient consultation and educational outreach. To this end, the Joslin Diabetes Center's Professional Education Department provides educational outreach to these PCPs, not just teaching new information, but fostering improved practice systems that integrate the diabetes care provided in the primary care setting with the regional services of the diabetes centers of excellence.

As a specialty center with national scope and singularity of focus, Joslin Diabetes Center is in a unique position to drive innovation in professional medical education in the prevention and treatment of diabetes and its related conditions and comorbidities. This key component of Joslin's mission is particularly important in the context of (1) the diabetes pandemic and its economic implications, (2) the treatment of most people with this condition in the primary care setting with insufficient numbers of endocrinologists and other expert staff to provide care for all, and (3) the lack of a national, optimized diabetes healthcare delivery framework for diabetes prevention, early diagnosis, treatment, and reduction of complication risk that ties all these healthcare components together. Further, national healthcare reform and the shift to quality-based reimbursements, Accountable Care Organizations (ACOs), and other constructs such as the Patient-Centered Medical Home and Pay for Performance, make it imperative that we begin to systematize diabetes care now.

While "traditional" CME such as lectures, meetings, and print and Web publications can produce measurable improvement in individual practitioner knowledge [16], less data support the effectiveness of CME as a performance improvement (PI) tool [17]. This finding is not surprising because the original mission of CME was not to measure performance improvement or clinical outcomes [18]. However, in today's environment, a focus on actual improvements in practice process and patient outcomes is crucial to worthwhile CME and is at the core of Joslin's effort to extend quality diabetes care to all practice settings.

A first step in linking traditional CME directly to PI is to design programs that provide physicians and clinical professionals with an accurate, guided tool to assess their own gaps in knowledge, competence, skill, and performance, which then enables them to engage in self-directed learning [19] – a critical component of an efficient, successful, targeted PI program [20]. It has been demonstrated that *unguided* individual physician self-assessments are inaccurate when compared to actual performance measures [20], and further research indicates that those who perform most poorly are the most likely to overestimate their abilities [21]. Further, clinicians may gravitate toward topics with which they are already familiar and avoid areas where they do not have as much experience [22–24], thereby missing an opportunity to gain perspective about their individual educational gaps. Thus, the Joslin system guides clinicians through a self-assessment process that we believe leads to a realistic targeting of areas for potential improvement.

The Institute of Medicine's (IOM) 2001 *Quality Chasm* report [25] acknowledged that health care in the new millennium should be knowledge-based, patient-centered, and systems-minded. Among other aligned changes, on January 1, 2005, the American Medical Association (AMA) approved guidelines by which up to 20 *AMA PRA Category 1 Credits*™ could be awarded for participation in structured performance improvement CME (PI-CME) activities (Fig. 13.2).

The foundation of Joslin's innovative CME program is known as the Joslin Professional Education Continuum (JPEC), which promotes continuous performance improvement (CPI) over time through CME learning activities both live and online (www.jpec.joslin.org) and via data-driven individual performance improvement (PI-CME) pathways. The approach is not "CME as a commodity," something the physician must "go to get," but one of CME integrated into everyday practice, contributing to the knowledge, competence, and skills necessary to improve both the quality of care provided and actual patient outcomes. Through "patient"-based interactions such as the Joslin Virtual Clinic, learners follow a patient through multiple visits while making clinical decisions. Point-of-care support materials are available (Joslin CareKit), providing downloadable materials to improve knowledge and competence, and also provide instruction in overcoming system barriers and addressing adherence issues.

Stage A: Baseline assessment of current practice performance
Assessment of current practice performance is conducted utilizing a specific performance measure[1] or set of measures that is applied to chart reviews, database queries, claims data, or another appropriate, predefined mechanism. Participating physicians must be actively involved in data collection and analysis and ideally will be provided with feedback comparing their performance to national benchmarks and to the performance of peers.

Stage B: Identification, design, and implementation of a practice improvement intervention
Based on the assessment of current practice deficits as identified in Stage A, a practice improvement intervention is designed and implemented. The design of the intervention should define the number of patients and the time required to assess the impact of the performance change. The implementation of the practice improvement is tracked using a predefined database, flow-sheet, or patient registry. [16]

Stage C: Reassessment of practice performance
After an appropriate, predetermined interval and using the performance measures adopted in Stage A, the effectiveness of the completed intervention is compared with the outcomes from Stage B. To complete this stage of the activity, physicians must summarize all three stages, including the clinical impact—if any—of the intervention, barriers to change, and lessons learned.

Fig. 13.2   Components of a complete performance improvement-CME activity

These activities are organized within JPEC's therapeutically focused Clinical Centers.[1] Learners access JPEC online via targeted direct messaging; participation in live activities aligned with one of the Clinical Centers; or via original or abstracted audio, Web, or mobile education (including the custom Joslin smart phone app). From each activity, the learner is then "pulled through" a Web-enabled Performance Improvement Pathway. Each structured Performance Improvement Pathway is designed to (1) use our guided system to help physicians identify gaps in their practice performance, (2) utilize recommended interventions to address those gaps, (3) reassess their progress, and (4) document resulting performance improvement. Thus, JPEC provides a roadmap for continuous quality improvement (CQI), allowing the physician to explore and identify individualized areas of improvement and contribute to better practice overall.

Research demonstrates that passive approaches to learning are ineffective in changing physician behavior [17]. JPEC is designed as a learning continuum of multifaceted activities combining several interventions and is based on data supporting the efficacy of this approach [23, 26]. The longitudinal design of our performance improvement includes underlying PI pathways and tools that exist over time, for a minimum of 3 years, while the knowledge and competence-based activities that feed them evolve and are updated regularly. This approach provides a foundation

---

[1] Four Clinical Centers have structured PI-CME activities. As of September 2010, *Type 2 Diabetes: Improving Office Systems of Care* and *Insulin Therapy* are approved through the American Board of Internal Medicine's (ABIM) Approved Quality Improvement (AQI) Pathway and are eligible for 20 points toward the Self-Evaluation of Practice Performance requirement of Maintenance of Certification (MOC). The remaining two activities are in the submission process at this writing.

of measurable data points integrated alongside each of the educational interventions. We believe that this will help us follow learners through the continuum, track performance change over time, and ultimately draw a straight line from the activities integrated within this approach to improved patient and population outcomes [27]. The data collected from this effort will help identify quality gaps in the primary care management of diabetes, drive the development of other integrated PI-CME programs, and improve the care of people with diabetes and related comorbidities.

In today's environment, any innovative CME program is incomplete without a thoughtful decision regarding sources of funding. Joslin's approach to "moving the needle" in diabetes care through CME is intensive, and funding sources are a vital component of the ultimate success of the JPEC system. (The reality is that the savings we have documented do not accrue to us or other programs that have produced them.) Joslin accepts commercial support from industry for our CME program, with additional safeguards above and beyond those needed for full ACCME compliance. To forestall any potential or perceived commercial bias, we utilize a collective funding approach to the overall development of JPEC activities. Each new commercially supported activity is designed to complement and leverage the resources of existing activities and support materials within each Clinical Center, effecting a pooled funding approach from multiple sources of support.

We therefore see JPEC as the final step in Joslin's process of promulgating optimal diabetes treatment by its:

1. Providing a physician-centric but practice-focused, longitudinal set of educational interventions intended to address the issues associated with individualized self-assessment of clinical gaps [20–24, 27, 28].
2. Promoting permanent behavior change by having learners cycle through a continuum of discovery, knowledge, competence, and performance domains.

This process starts with Joslin Clinic in Boston, an evolving state-of-the-art diabetes center of excellence practice model that we continually refine. It next moves to our Affiliates, regionalizing the specialty model. Finally, through outreach such as the Professional Education efforts centered on JPEC and the regional influence of the affiliates program, we seek to impact the primary care practices where most people with diabetes receive their care. This is a work in progress, and undoubtedly, as we evolve, and the healthcare delivery system environment changes as well, we will, in concert, provide a more effective, systematized approach to the care of people with diabetes throughout the nation. Stay tuned!

Editor's comments: The Joslin team's improvement project leverages provider and patient education to optimize care and support superior outcomes for this costly and devastating disease. But beyond this they have incorporated provider self-assessment and performance tracking methods. They make extensive use of nonphysician professionals, including nurse educators, and have developed complimentary roles for primary physicians and diabetes specialists in providing care across the broad disease population with variable severity and needs. They understand the true complexity of diabetes care and have taken on the challenges. These themes will be repeated often in the chapters that follow. (JTH)

References

1. Woodwell DA, Cherry DK. National ambulatory medical care survey: 2002 summary. Advance data from vital and health statistics; no. 346. Hyattsville: National Center for Health Statistics. 2004. http://www.cdc.gov/nchs/data/ad/ad346.pdf. Accessed 26 Jan 2007.
2. Rosamond W, Fegal K, Friday G, et al. on behalf of the American Heart Association. Heart disease and stroke statistics: 2007. Circulation. 2007;115:e69–71.
3. Resnick HE, Foster GL, Bardsley J, Ratner RE. Achievement of American Diabetes Association clinical practice recommendations among U.S. adults with diabetes, 1999–2002: the national health and nutrition examination survey (NHANES). Diabetes Care. 2006;29:531–7.
4. Centers for Disease Control and Prevention. National diabetes fact sheet: general information and national estimates on diabetes in the United States. Atlanta: U.S. Department of Health and Human Services, Centers for Disease Control and Prevention; 2007. p. 2008.
5. American Diabetes Association Web site. http://www.diabetes.org/diabetes-basics/diabetes-statistics/?utm_source=WWW&utm_medium=DropDownDB&utm_content=Statistics&utm_campaign=CON. Accessed 17 Dec 2010.
6. Spann SJ, Nutting PA, Galliher JM, et al. Management of type 2 diabetes in the primary care setting: a practice-based research network study. Ann Fam Med. 2006;4(1):23–31.
7. Parchman ML, Romero RL, Pugh JA. Encounters by patients with type 2 diabetes – complex and demanding: an observational study. Ann Fam Med. 2006;4(1):40–5.
8. Resnick HE, Foster GL, Bardsley J, Ratner RE. Achievement of American Diabetes Association clinical practice recommendations among U.S. adults with diabetes, 1999–2002: the national health and nutrition examination survey (NHANES). Diabetes Care. 2006;29:531–7.
9. Brown JB, Nichols GA. Slow response to loss of glycemic control in type 2 diabetes mellitus. Am J Manag Care. 2003;9:213–7.
10. Beaser R, Okeke E, Neighbours J, Brown J, Ronk K, Wolyniec WW. Coordinated primary and specialty care for type 2 diabetes, guidelines and systems: an educational needs assessment. Endocr Pract. 2011;17:1–26.
11. Klein R, Klein BE, Moss SE, Cruickshanks KJ. The Wisconsin Epidemiologic Study of Diabetic Retinopathy: XVII. The 14-year incidence and progression of diabetic retinopathy and associated risk factors in type 1 diabetes. Ophthalmology. 1998;105:1799–800.
12. American Diabetes Association. Economic costs of diabetes in the U.S. in 2007. Diabetes Care. 2008;31:596–615.
13. The Diabetes Control and Complications Trial Research Group. The Effect of intensive treatment of diabetes on the development and progression of long-term complications in insulin-dependent diabetes mellitus. N Engl J Med. 1993;329:977–86.
14. UK Prospective Diabetes Study Group. Association of glycaemia with macrovascular and microvascular complications of type 2 diabetes (UKPDS 35). BMJ. 2000;321:405–12.
15. Lloyd-Jones D, Adams RJ, Brown TM, et al. on behalf of the American Heart Association Statistics Committee and Stroke Statistics Subcommittee. Heart disease and stroke statistics 2010 update. a report from the American Heart Association. Circulation. 2010;121:e46–215.
16. Hager M, Russell S, Fletcher SW, editors. Continuing education in the health professions: improving healthcare through lifelong learning. In: Proceedings of a conference sponsored by the Josiah Macy Jr. foundation, 28 Nov–1 Dec 2007, Bermuda. New York: Josiah Macy, Jr. Foundation; 2008. http://josiahmacyfoundation.org/docs/macy_puns/pub_ContEd_inHealth-Prof.pdf. Accessed 24 Sept 2011.
17. Davis DA, Thomson MA, Oxman AD, Haynes RB. Changing physician performance. A systematic review of the effect of continuing medical education strategies. JAMA. 1995;274:700–5.
18. Dorman T. Response to "reform of CME" published in JAMA. SACME. 2009;22:1–2.
19. Colthart I, Bagnall G, Evans A, et al. The effectiveness of self-assessment on the identification of learner needs learner activity, and impact on clinical practice: BEME Guide no. 10. Med Teach. 2008;30(2):124.

20. Davis DA, Mazmanian PE, Fordis M, Van Harrison R, Thorpe KE, Perrier L. Accuracy of physician self-assessment compared with observed measures of competence: a systematic review. JAMA. 2006;296(9):1094–102.
21. Kruger J, Dunning D. Unskilled and unaware of it: how difficulties in recognizing one's own incompetence lead to inflated self-assessments. J Pers Soc Psychol. 1999;77(6):1121–34.
22. Sibley JC, Sackett DL, Neufeld V, Gerrard B, Rudnick KV, Fraser W. A randomized trial of continuing medical education. N Engl J Med. 1982;306(9):511.
23. Duffy FD, Holmboe ES. Self-assessment in lifelong learning and improving performance in practice. JAMA. 2006;296:1137–9.
24. Eva KW, Regehr G. Self-assessment in the health professions: a reformulation and research agenda. Acad Med. 2005;80(10 Suppl):S81–4.
25. Committee on Quality of Health Care in America, Institute of Medicine. Crossing the quality chasm: a new health system for the 21st century. Washington: National Academy Press; 2001.
26. Grimshaw JM, Thomas RE, MacLennan G, et al. Effectiveness and efficiency of guideline dissemination and implementation strategies. Health Technol Assess. 2004;8:iii–iv, 1–72.
27. Institute of Medicine (IOM). Redesigning continuing education in the health professions. Washington: The National Academies Press; 2010.
28. Institute of Medicine (IOM). To err is human: building a safer health system. Washington: National Academy Press; 2000.

Chapter 14
Osteoporosis: Breaking Bones Is Not Inevitable

Richard M. Dell

Keywords Kaiser • Osteoporosis • Fracture • Healthy Bones • Pyramid approach • Quality improvement • Population care • Shame and blame

When I finished my orthopedic surgery training at USC in 1987, I was faced with the choices of private practice, academics, or the Kaiser system. I chose Kaiser because of its integrated model of care and its commitment to using information technology to manage patients. Within Kaiser, I have never had to worry about variable reimbursement and conflicting financial priorities getting in the way of my providing necessary care and working with my colleagues to develop our osteoporosis fracture prevention program. *Fracture prevention makes sense in Kaiser because it is considerably less expensive to prevent a hip fracture than to manage it, simple as that.* Kaiser's state-of-the-art electronic medical record (EMR) also supports my patient care and clinical research (Fig. 14.1).

What Is the problem with Osteoporosis Care?

Osteoporosis is a disease of postmenopausal women and older people more generally that is characterized by loss of bone density and structure. This increases the risk of fractures for individual patients and the burden of fractures for our aging population.

When we discuss the current state of osteoporosis disease management, there is the bad news, the good news, as well as the sad news.

R.M. Dell, MD (✉)
Department of Orthopedics, Kaiser Permanente, Downey, CA, USA
e-mail: Richard.M.Dell@kp.org

J.T. Harrington and E.D. Newman (eds.), *Great Health Care: Making It Happen*,
DOI 10.1007/978-1-4614-1198-7_14, © Springer Science+Business Media, LLC 2012

Fig. 14.1 Rick Dell, suited up for redesigning osteoporosis care

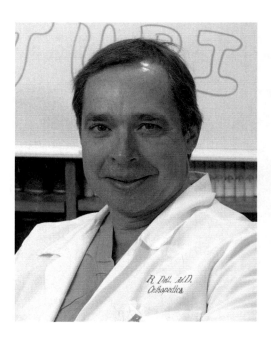

The *bad news* is that osteoporosis is a huge problem in the United States today with over nine million women and 2.8 million men afflicted and another 40 million men and women having low bone mass that has yet to reach the diagnostic threshold for osteoporosis [1]. These patients are all at increased risk for fragility fractures, and over two million experience new fractures every year, including 325,000 hip fractures [2]. Their total cost is over $18 billion a year in the USA. Hip fractures are of particular concern since more than 20% of these patients die within the year after they fracture. And beyond all this bad news, there is even worse news. The tsunami of 75 million baby boomers now starting to turn 65 will drastically increase the number of at-risk patients.

The *good news* is that these predictions are not inevitable. We now have bone density (DXA) scanners to help us identify patients who have osteoporosis and low bone mass, and we understand the other predictors of fracture risk. We have new fracture risk calculators that incorporate this information to estimate patients' fracture risk [3], and we have a wide assortment of medicines that can lower this risk by up to 50%. There are also excellent examples of osteoporosis disease management programs that identify, risk-stratify, treat, and then track patients. Kaiser's Healthy Bones Program and the Geisinger osteoporosis disease management program are just two of these within the United States that have in fact reduced their patients' fracture rates [4, 5].

The *sad news* is that today in the United States most patients will not see the benefits of what we know to do or a systematic approach to the management of their osteoporosis. The failure to attack this problem is related largely to the current reimbursement for fragments of care rather than coordinated care and favorable outcomes. In addition, clinicians are generally paid well for treating the fragility fractures, but poorly for preventing them.

The History of Kaiser's Healthy Bones Program

Let's turn the clock back to 1997 when a small team of clinicians, radiology technicians, and administrators came up with the idea of developing an osteoporosis and fracture prevention program at my medical center in Kaiser Bellflower in Southern California. I wish I could say we developed a beautiful systematic model of care with total consensus. We already had many of the pieces of an osteoporosis and fracture prevention program in place, but we could not agree initially on how to put all these pieces together, or even come up with a common goal. Some in our team wanted to develop a comprehensive osteoporosis education program to better teach the benefits of calcium and vitamin D to patients and clinicians. Others wanted to increase DXA use by putting up posters and sending out reminders for clinicians to order DXAs more effectively. And the majority of our team wanted to focus our attention on reducing the overall hip fracture rate at our hospital.

As an Orthopedic Surgeon, I had always been frustrated that the hip fracture patients I was treating could have avoided the problem if adequate measures had been taken prior to their fracturing. As such, I became the most vocal advocate of reducing our hip fracture rate by whatever means would prove to be necessary. I had already been tracking our hip fractures at Kaiser for several years using a database of all surgical procedures performed. The number of hip fractures had been increasing steadily over the previous 5 years, driven by Kaiser's growing population.

I convinced our team to set a goal of reducing the hip fracture rate at our hospital by 20% over the next 5 years. We then brainstormed on how we would use the fragmented pieces of our osteoporosis care and current resources with minimal – I really mean minimal – extra resources to:

1. Identify the individuals who were most likely to have a hip fracture in the next 5–10 years
2. Risk-stratify them into high, moderate, and low lower risk cohorts
3. Initiate treatment on the high-risk patients first before progressing to those at lower risk
4. Track our patients on treatment to ensure compliance
5. Develop monthly performance reports for both our program at the medical center, and for individual clinicians

It only took a few meetings to set our main objectives, but when it came to deciding how we would actually do the real work, our team developed "analysis paralysis." Too much time was being spent arguing over the perfect strategy for all patients instead of starting any real work. That's when we hit on the pyramid approach. We called this the pyramid approach because the pyramid went from the highest risk

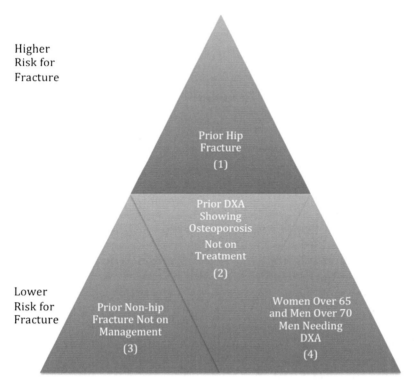

Fig. 14.2 The pyramid of risk for hip fracture. A serial approach to identifying and managing our at-risk populations from highest to lowest was critical to our success

group that had the least number of patients to progressively lower risk groups that were made up of more and more patients (Fig. 14.2).

1. We would focus first on the small number of patients that already had a hip fracture. Most of these patients just needed anti-osteoporosis treatment and a referral to our fall prevention class in physical therapy. A few would need a home health safety visit, and some would also need evaluation by our Endocrinologist.
2. We would next identify all patients who had a prior DXA scan that showed osteoporosis who were not already prescribed anti-osteoporosis treatment, or who were previously on treatment and had stopped. Our care manager initiated treatment and made referrals when appropriate.
3. We would then evaluate the nonhip fracture patients at highest risk of soon having a hip fracture, the over 65 population at high risk of falling, or with a previous fracture at another site. If the patient needed a DXA, we ordered the DXA and sent the results to our care manager and the patient's primary care clinician. If treatment was needed, our care manager initiated treatment, and then helped in the decisions for referral to PT, Home Health, endocrinology, or other departments.

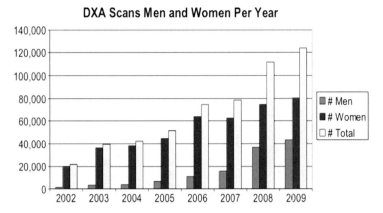

Fig. 14.3 DXA scans per year. Bone density measurements for patients at risk for osteoporosis have increased each year

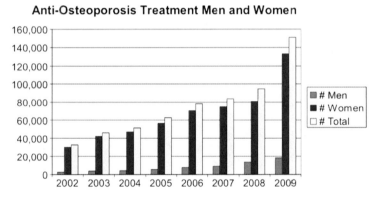

Fig. 14.4 Treating more patients with osteoporosis has decreased the number of fragility fractures in our at-risk patient populations

4. We would then focus on women over 65 and men over 70 years old who have not yet had a fracture or a DEXA scan. For them, we ordered the DXA and initiated appropriate treatment and referrals.

In taking this approach, we recognized that our goal of reducing hip fractures would only be achieved as we moved from the small population at the highest individual risk to the larger populations at lower risk. But our proceeding this way permitted us to learn and get good at our work without being overwhelmed at the outset.

The monthly and cumulative reports that showed how many patients in each of these four groups were receiving bone density measurement (Fig. 14.3) and anti-osteoporosis treatment (Fig. 14.4) were key to the success of the program. It kept our team focused on the actual work that was getting done or was still needed. Now our team meetings had everyone giving feedback about their piece of the program and a systematic approach to problem solving quickly developed. The utilization of our DXA scanner quickly improved, the number of patients appropriately getting anti-osteoporosis medication quickly improved, the fall reduction and osteoporosis education classes were revamped and improved, and most importantly, after 2 years we started to see a decrease in our hip fracture rates.

Our osteoporosis and fracture prevention program needed a catchy name that reflects our focus. Initially, we used the Hip At Risk Program (HARP). I though HARP was the perfect name because for many years I harped to anyone who would listen that our HARP was a model of care we could use not just for osteoporosis, but for any disease management program. Just identify the population at risk, risk stratify that group, start with the group at highest risk, and systematically work the list to treat and then track those on treatment – again not rocket science! Several years later, we changed our name to the Healthy Bones Program, but I'm still harping!

Good Research Design – No. Good Patient Care – Yes

We could have done a beautifully designed research project where all the variables were set and patients were divided into treatment and nontreatment groups. But instead we choose a completely different approach, a continuous quality improvement project that reorganized and coordinated the pieces of our existing program. We decided quickly what worked and what didn't work. Instead of studying care, we were learning by studying while doing. We also felt having a group of patients in the nontreatment group was unacceptable.

Please don't get me wrong, good research is important, but our team was making changes to our program extremely rapidly, and …

… in my mind what was lacking in the literature were examples of successful disease management programs on real-world populations. We already knew that DXAs were great at identifying patients with osteoporosis; we already knew that treatment decreases hip fracture rates by up to 50%. What we didn't know was whether we could really put the pieces of care together to develop a program that could systematically identify a huge population of patients at risk for osteoporosis and hip fractures, and quickly close the care gaps in their treatment.

So what do we do differently than the way most osteoporosis and fracture care is done in the USA today? We developed a monthly work list for our clinicians and care managers with specific recommendations for how to close the care gaps. We systematically started with the patients we considered at the highest risk of having a hip fracture and progressive worked our way through the list. We supported our providers' care of individual patients by reducing their work of coordinating care and putting them in a position to use their time to greatest advantage.

If you are thinking to yourself "That's not rocket science," well you are exactly right. We all make our individual work lists. The power is in teams doing the same. Sometimes the simplest ideas are the most effective. In fact, our ideas on disease management were quickly picked up by the rest of the medical centers in Kaiser Southern California, as well as most medical centers eventually in the Kaiser system.

Population Care, a Continuous Improvement Team, and Improving Results

So how have we done in Kaiser Southern California with this basic model? Does a 37% plus reduction in the expected number of hip fractures sound like an effective program? I think so considering that the medications have around a 50% reduction in hip fracture ra e in controlled studies, and many of the other therapies like calcium, vitamin D, fall reduction classes, balance classes, and patient education also help. But we thought we could do better still, and in fact our 37% reduction has been progressively improving as we do a better and better job at identifying patients most likely to have a hip fracture, getting them evaluated, started on and adherent to appropriate medicines, and provided the other appropriate therapies shown to decrease the hip fracture rate.

Are we content with our results? No. We are constantly reevaluating ways to better manage our patients. Weekly teleconferences and quarterly face-to-face meeting with our Healthy Bones Team help reinforce what works and doesn't work. We now provide monthly performance reports to all our medical centers in Kaiser Southern California. Our reports are really good, and no one can accuse us of not having the data. Our EMRs inform our coordinators about exactly who is having a fracture, who is getting a DEXA and/or treatment, and who is staying on treatment.

I personally think there is nothing like competition to drive improvement. Most people are competitive, and those in the medical field are some of the most competitive of all people. All we really needed to do to see improvement was to show that one medical center was not doing as well as another medical center. Some call it shame and blame some call it a great way to minimizing variation; I call it the most effective way of stimulating folks to get the work done – basically you get a list and you work the list.

Can we replicate the same ideas elsewhere as effectively as we did at Kaiser? Absolutely! In fact, there are programs at Geisinger, the Fracture Liaison Services in the UK and Canada, and others that identify patients at highest risk for hip fractures and get them treated. Interestingly, their successful approaches look just like ours. So I believe that we know what to do and how to do it. What gives some health systems an advantage over most is supportive leadership and a financial environment that supports teamwork and integration of care.

Implications for United States Health Policy

I'm praying folks from the policy side of Medicare will read this, since we could start the journey of reducing the hip fracture rate in the USA, if others follow the ten relatively easy steps we have used (see below) and are rewarded for their successes. I'm even willing to make a wager with Don Berwick, the current head of the Centers for Medicare and Medicaid Services (CMS), or whoever is his successor at CMS. The wager is simple: I bet you I can lower the current hip fracture rate in the USA by 25% at a lower cost than it would take to care for their hip fractures. In real terms, that means roughly 75,000 fewer hip fractures per year than expected.

I pray as well that the folks who are opposing U.S. healthcare reform will reconsider and come to understand the opportunities we have for doing better at a lower cost. This is a win-win-win situation. The patients win since a hip fracture is a devastating condition with a high complication rate and high death rate. The medical community wins since resources are utilized more efficiently and at a lower cost. Society wins because less money is being spent. There is one more win. I will have won my wager with the folks at CMS!

A ten-step guide for building a fragility fracture prevention program:

1. Strong champion(s) are required
   I cannot overemphasize the importance of one or more strong champions to cement the Healthy Bones Team together. Without a champion to guide a goal-focused team, you will fail. The same is true for practice or health system leadership that supports champions and the improvement team. I eat my Wheaties every morning!

2. Set an achievable goal and start working
   The Team will do what it takes to drive a 20–25% reduction in the hip fracture rate while working within its budget if an ambitious but realistic goal is defined.

3. Identify your patients at risk for a hip fracture
   The key point is having an effective method of identifying the populations who have experienced hip and other fragility fractures, and later the others who have yet to fracture. EMRs and registries are particularly helpful, but just a list of CPT bills sent out is a nice starting point and one that Medicare could use if it decides to implement a Healthy Bones Program at a national level.

4. Risk-stratify your population
   Risk-stratify patients into those who need DEXA scan and/or treatment, starting with the highest risk patients for having a hip fracture. This can also be based on age, sex, race, type of fracture, BMI, prior treatment, and some type of fracture risk score such as FRAX that can be calculated with or without a T-score [3]. You can call the highest risk patients "the big bang for the buck patients" since they are most likely to have a hip fracture, and it doesn't take evaluating and treating many of them to prevent a hip fracture. At the other end of the risk spectrum are a larger group of patients at lower risk, but with a higher number of fractures in aggregate.

5. Create work lists of those who need DEXA and/or treatment
   Send a monthly (ideally a real-time) report of those patients who need a DEXA and/or treatment to care managers who will actually order the DEXA and/or initiate treatment. Getting the right data to the right person at the right time is crucial. We have just-in-time nurse practitioner rule-driven clinics to evaluate each patient immediately after a DEXA scan, to get the DEXA read, the patient treated, the necessary labs done, the consults sent, and the education given all at one sitting.

6. Measure how everyone is doing and study the variations

   A monthly report of how each medical center and region compares to other medical centers and regions should be used to encourage improvement. Competition is good; it drives constant improvement and helps to minimize variation of care. Standardizing care first makes it easier to move the dial higher.

7. Keep what works and share best ideas

   Track how well your program is doing over time, and constantly re-evaluate what is working and what is not. The best-performing medical centers can share ideas and best practices with those medical centers that are struggling. This is how rapid cycle process improvement is used in business instead of a randomized controlled study with fixed protocols. If an idea works then share it, and if an idea fails, either fix it or scrap it, but learn from the failures. "Perfection is the enemy of the good."

8. Provide incentives for good and best performance

   Sometimes it is good to offer financial rewards for performance. Also the potential of holding back full payments for managing a hip or other fragility fracture if the osteoporosis and fall assessment is not done has been discussed. At this point, most programs are using carrots, but I think the sticks may not be that far away. Just knowing you are the best is a stronger motivator than any monetary reward for many clinicians, and most clinicians will say they didn't train for all those years to be mediocre; they trained to be the best.

9. Measure reductions in relation to expected hip fracture rates

   The reduction in hip fracture is based on age/sex/race-adjusted hip fracture risk in each age/sex/race category in your area. This is relatively easy to do at Kaiser and also easy at regional, state, and national levels. Within local health systems, a comparison to baseline fracture number each subsequent year may be sufficient. It takes a minimum of a year or two to see significant changes, but the hip fracture rates will begin to decrease if you get the high-risk patients on medication.

10. Keep setting the bar higher

    Look for long-term trends of reduction in hip fracture rates. A 20–25% reduction in the hip fracture rate should be an initial goal. But don't stop if you're lucky enough to hit the 25% reduction goal; just reset your goal to a higher benchmark. The constant cycling of improvements in the Healthy Bones Program reinforces the idea that you are on a journey and not heading to a destination.

Editor's comments: Rick Dell is a leader in improving quality of care for this important, under-managed disease. He is an orthopedic surgeon who took responsibility earlier than most of his colleagues for preventing fragility fractures, not just treating them. His team has leveraged the Kaiser information technology resources, their culture of team care, and an integrated business model into the best care for osteoporosis anywhere in the U.S – and they have the data to show it. Kaiser has a strong commitment to the patient centered medical home, but like other integrated systems, they have recognized that high performing chronic disease management requires inclusive, system-based, specialized programs. His example in Kaiser Southern California has driven broad improvement in post-fracture care across the Kaiser system. JTH

References

1. Prevalence report. National Osteoporosis Foundation. http://www.nof.org/advocacy/resources/prevalencereport. Accessed 20 April 2011.
2. Burge R, Dawson-Hughes B, Solomon DH, Wong JB, King A, Tosteson A. Incidence and economic burden of osteoporosis-related fractures in the United States, 2005–2025. J Bone Miner Res. 2007;22:465–75.
3. Dawson-Hughes B on behalf of the National Osteoporosis Foundation Guide Committee. FRAX bone treatment algorithm: a revised clinician's guide to the prevention and treatment of osteoporosis – commentary. J Clin Endocrinol Metab. 2008;93:2463–5. http://www.natap.org/2008/HIV/071508_07.htm. Accessed 20 April 2011.
4. Dell R, Greene D, Schelkun SR, Williams K. Osteoporosis disease management: the role of the orthopedic surgeon. J Bone Joint Surg (Am). 2008;90:188–94.
5. Newman E. A schema for effective osteoporosis management: outcomes of the Geisinger Health System Osteoporosis Program. Dis Manage Health Outcomes. 2003;11:611–6.

Chapter 15
Rheumatoid Arthritis: Diagnose Early and Treat to Target

John J. Cush

Keywords Rheumatoid arthritis- • Treat to target • Personalized medicine • Diagnose early • Treat aggressively • DMARD • Disease activity measurement • RAPID3 • CDAI • GAS

"If we keep doing what we're doing, we're gonna keep getting what we got."

Yogi Berra

In January 1970 we arrived at the hospital early to ensure a meeting with the physician to receive an update or word of hope. My dad was ill with metastatic cancer, and recent events indicated he was on the downhill slide. Hope now rested in test and imaging results and interpretations from the rounding physician. We waited bedside most of that snowy day, and finally the white coat healer arrived with the medical chart. Pages were turned, results reviewed, a stethoscope brandished, and then the all-knowing soother nodded, mumbled and left after few minutes. The brevity of it all left us silenced and troubled. Much was wrong, but little was said to the patient or family. While this may have been routine care, it was lacking. At that moment, I knew I could be a physician, because I cared more and was a better communicator, even as a 10th grade high school student.

Fast forward to 1985, the second year of my rheumatology fellowship at UT Southwestern Medical School and Parkland Memorial Hospital. My mentor and chairman Dr. Peter Lipsky guided me into clinical trials research of nonsteroidal anti-inflammatory drugs (NSAIDs) and biologic agents for rheumatoid arthritis (RA). This work added standardized data gathering and outcome assessments to my routine patient care, and changed my approach forever. I came to recognize that great advances were as likely to result from practice improvements as from new pharmaceuticals, and that falling into unchanging routines was contrary to such advances.

In the great song "As good as I once was", country artist Toby Keith laments the waning of his prowess and verve with ageing. Fortunately for physicians (and our patients), we often gain experience, knowledge and insight with maturation. Mentoring by teachers, peers and patients leads us to understand the unknown, meet the needs of our patients, and inspire others in return. I believe that all physicians strive to deliver personalized medical care based on attentive observation and sound medical intervention. However, these goals

J.J. Cush (✉)
Baylor University Medical Center, Dallas, TX, USA
e-mail: jjcush@gmail.com

J.T. Harrington and E.D. Newman (eds.), *Great Health Care: Making it Happen*, DOI 10.1007/978-1-4614-1198-7_15, © Springer Science+Business Media, LLC 2012 *may fall victim to the "routine", causing physicians to fall short of providing what is great and necessary. The enemies of change and innovation include limited time, income expectations, insufficient renewal of knowledge, and low motivation.*

Experience has taught me that it's not enough to be efficient, productive, and skilled. My patients and their problems have challenged me to integrate the rigor and detail of clinical trial metrics into my medical practice, and then to share these processes with my colleagues.

John J. Cush

New treatments have multiplied in the last three decades that improve rheumatologists' capabilities for altering and even controlling RA. More recently, we have recognized that new approaches to providing these discoveries will also be required if RA patients are to realize their benefits, including:

• Early diagnosis and early treatment,
• Sensitive and practical RA disease activity measurements to direct treatment,
• Accelerating treatment until inflammation in the joints and other tissues is controlled, known in our field as "Treating to Target", and
• Providing personalized patient care, because RA is variable from one patient to another. Not only do responses to treatment and side effects vary, but patients differ in their preferences and priorities for disease management.

This chapter will discuss others' and my work in improving these aspects of care through developing and testing new processes. Process testing is now the standard in our practice and in those of a growing number of colleagues. I will also share the results of a series of surveys I've conducted to learn how other rheumatologists are practicing and why. Positive change requires time and work. Rheumatology is in the process of changing – one foot anchored in the past, and the other stepping toward the future.

The Earlier the Better

A group of Canadian researchers interviewed a large number of leaders in musculoskeletal medicine regarding emerging changes in arthritis care [1]. They identified 5 main models being used to deliver care for RA: (1) Specialized arthritis programs delivering comprehensive, multidisciplinary team care; (2) triage of patients with musculoskeletal conditions by primary physicians to the appropriate services, including rheumatology specialty care; and (3) ongoing primary care RA management in collaboration with a consultant rheumatologist. Two further models were suggested to address issues relating to rural access: (4) rural consultation support, and (5) telemedicine. Improving access to care was in the forefront of their discussions and recommendations.

The best way to eradicate diseases is to prevent them in the first place; however, this requires understandings of cause(s) and pathophysiology that are currently lacking for many, like cancers, diabetes, hypertension, and RA. In these cases, early diagnosis and treatment becomes central to minimizing disease impacts. This approach limits the harm inflicted by acute disorders such as bacterial pneumonia or tissue infections, alters the course and outcomes for chronic disorders such as RA and diabetes, and can increasingly change once-lethal disorders into chronic controllable diseases, such as HIV and some leukemias.

RA afflicts 1.3 million people in the USA. They will suffer and even die prematurely if they are not diagnosed and treated early and optimally. The obvious effects of the disease are pain, disability, and impaired quality of life, but it doesn't stop here. Until recently, those afflicted might expect a shortened life span by 10 years, a 60% chance of work disability after 10 years of disease, and an increased lifetime risk for cancers (twofold), cardiovascular disease (two to threefold), and serious infections (six to ninefold) [2]. Optimal management of RA can now limit these long-term consequences.

During the mid 1980s, my early research focused on clinical trials of new drugs and the underlying disease mechanisms operating in RA, immunopathogenesis in a big word. During that era, the "early diagnosis and aggressive treatment of RA" was advocated by a small number of rheumatologist investigators, even though the treatments then fell short of what is available today. We learned that the inception events in RA included vascular changes, antigen-driven mononuclear cell inflammation, and later a dysregulated, self-amplifying cascade of destructive inflammatory molecules. We describe these events to our patients now as something causing the body's immune system to become overactive that triggers a persistent, destructive inflammatory reaction in the joint linings and other tissues, the same reactions that our bodies mount to heal wounds and fight infections – except in RA they don't shut down. These inception events usually begin many months before the patient experiences the onset of typical symptoms – pain, stiffness, and swelling. Even with prompt diagnosis, they will direct a long and destructive process – unless they are interrupted.

Rheumatologists recognize the gravity of this challenge and have uniformly, willfully, and widely adopted the mantra for RA to "diagnose early and treat aggressively." A wealth of instructive research has shown that:

1. The earlier a disease-modifying anti-rheumatic drug (DMARD) or biologic therapy directed against specific inflammatory reactions is initiated, the better the long-term outcomes. The converse is equally and dreadfully true – that delays of as little as 4 months lead to poorer clinical outcomes and irrevocable damage to tissues.
2. All DMARD therapies work best when used early.
3. Early RA is defined as "the earlier, the better," although most rheumatologists prefer to diagnose patients and treat within 12 weeks of symptom onset.
4. Patients who are at high risk for more aggressive disease can often be identified early based on clinical, laboratory, and radiographic assessments, and with time, these indicators become even clearer (Table 15.1).
5. And sadly, significant delays beyond 4 months still exist in referral to rheumatology, and less than 15% of all RA patients are seen within the first 6 months of their illness. In my surveys of US rheumatologists, the average wait to see a rheumatologist is 38 work days, only 27% of patients have a new appointment

Table 15.1 Poor prognostic predictors in early RA

Clinical features
- High disease activity: Many swollen joints, a high disease activity score
- Extra-articular manifestations: rheumatoid nodules, Sjogren's syndrome (inflammation in glands that produce tears and saliva), Felty's syndrome (destruction of blood cells), neuropathy

Disability
- Functional surveys such as the Health Assessment Questionnaire (HAQ) showing progressive impairment

Laboratory features
- High titer serum rheumatoid factor or anti-CCP antibodies
- High tests for inflammation: C-reactive protein or ESR

Imaging
- Erosions on joint X-rays, ultrasound, or MRI

wait time that is less than 2 weeks, and for 40%, the average wait is 5 weeks to 6 months. Not only are patients referred too late, but they may then be provided a next available rheumatology appointment weeks or months down the road.

Nonetheless, all rheumatologists I know are fully committed to providing immediate consultative care to any "early arthritis" patient referred for this reason by their primary care colleagues, because this is when treatment is most successful. If only this happened more often. It's not surprising that the vast majority of early arthritis patients first seek medical evaluations from their primary care physicians (PCPs); however, the majority of these patients are not promptly referred. Most observational studies show that RA makes up only 1–2% of new PCP visits. Despite the gravity of early RA in the rheumatologist's mind, it is a low priority and an easily overlooked condition in primary care. RA patients are "needles in the haystack" among many others with similar and confusing joint and muscle symptoms that present to primary physicians. And its gradual onset may convince many RA patients that their symptoms are nothing serious.

Once they present to their PCP, most early RA patients experience time-consuming diagnostic tests, overreliance on palliative therapies including nonsteroidal anti-inflammatory drugs (NSAIDs) and steroids, and referral delays. PCPs seldom examine the patient for the simple symptoms and signs of early arthritis validated by British rheumatologist Paul Emery: more than 30 min morning stiffness in the joints, and/or 2 or more swollen joints, and/or pain with squeezing the joints of the mid-hand and forefoot. Test results are often normal or negative in the first 6 months after the onset of RA, but PCPs are not taught any of this during their training. On the other hand, PCPs commonly point to overburdened and insufficient local rheumatology workforces.

In fact, early consultation, diagnosis, and use of DMARD therapy occur most frequently when there is immediate and ongoing cooperative care between the PCP and the rheumatologist. I assert that rheumatologists should be appropriately used to meet the need for early diagnosis and intervention in RA, and that this requires teamwork. Rheumatologists need to provide timely access to care and educate their referring physicians as to who should be referred, when, and how urgently, and primary physicians need to listen up rather than continuing to do what they learned in training. For most rheumatologists, the diagnosis of arthritis is usually expedient, expert, and based on clinical rather than laboratory evidence. When challenged, they affirm that "greater than 80% of all diagnoses are made in the first 90 s of a new patient visit." This is not unlike other disciplines where experience and insight lend to facile diagnoses based on pattern recognition and clinical findings of high predictive value.

To better understand this challenge, I researched and coauthored a textbook on early RA, with a focus on early drug intervention and the positive results derived from early RA clinics in Europe [3]. I learned that despite their firm support of the "diagnose early, treat aggressively" paradigm, US rheumatologists were doing little to change referral patterns and access to care in their daily practices. My partners and I assessed approaches being used by others to improve access for our early inflammatory arthritis patients. We then tested three different models of new patient evaluation before deciding on the best course for our practice:

1. *Free arthritis screening clinics:* Working with the hospital public relations department, we promoted several "free arthritis screening clinics" which ran on a Tuesday afternoon every 3–4 months and were staffed by two to three rheumatologists and a nurse practitioner. Most patients were recruited from newspaper advertisements and local announcements. Each patient filled out a half page survey form including their primary complaint, past medical history, current medications, and a symptom review. Physicians and a nurse or study coordinator evaluated each patient and completed a one-page evaluation form. Patients were provided copies of the evaluation form, referral guidance, or a future appointment with the rheumatologist's practice when appropriate. We ran four of these clinics and were able to see over 60 patients during each.

   The Bottom line. Very few early RA patients were identified, but all of the rheumatologists were enthralled with providing satisfying consultative services and decisive proper placements for future care. This program was also modestly useful in recruiting patients to our osteoarthritis and RA clinical trials.

2. *Early Arthritis Screening Clinic.* We promoted a weekly Tuesday afternoon "Early Arthritis Clinic" with a one page "Dear Doctor" letter and a form for "early arthritis" patient referral to over 200 primary care and orthopedic physicians, promising to see all referrals within 2 weeks. Our letter detailed the need for early diagnosis and treatment of RA and the rules for referral promoted by Paul Emery, as outlined above. A rheumatologist, nurse practitioner, and internal medicine resident staffed each clinic. After 1 year, we were only seeing four to five new referrals per week, only 10% had early inflammatory arthritis, and those found to actually have inflammatory arthritis had had symptoms ranging from 16–52 weeks.

   The Bottom Line. Promotion of our early arthritis clinic and the need for early referral was only modestly successful. Our outreach resonated with a minority of physicians. Over time, this program was morphed from an early arthritis referral clinic to an "any arthritis" referral clinic. We provided useful services, but were still only seeing one to two new RA patients every 3 months, many fewer than we believed to be present in our health system's population.

3. *Network-wide Early Arthritis Clinics.* We learned from our past failures by doing more of the same on a larger scale. We recruited nine local rheumatologists who committed to providing rapid patient evaluation and used the hospital network to promote these early RA consult services. A centralized referral phone number was established. Repeated announcements and reminders were sent to all physicians in the network, who provided care collectively to almost two million people. This program brought us some patients, but hardly the numbers of new RA patients we projected.

   The Bottom Line. Insufficient results stemmed from the variable commitment by both the participating rheumatologists and the referring physicians who were more interested in referring joint complaint patients without restriction. To develop a large scale, regional early arthritis network requires a full commitment by an institution or community and all practitioners. It requires ongoing education, promotion, and coordinated transfer of patients and their records, none of which are easily or cheaply achieved.

Research on creating early referral and access has suggested other methods as well, including: (1) Physician-to-Physician requests for expedited consultation – great intentions, but seldom if ever performed; (2) Prescreening and chart review of early arthritis referrals; (3) Screening algorithms or surveys – population-based tools that allow patients or PCPs to know when they may have RA and should see a rheumatologist; or (4) use of physician extenders to screen and evaluate all new referrals [4].

To diagnose early and treat RA aggressively, I've concluded the following:

1. Patients with new-onset arthritis want an expert evaluation and prompt relief of their symptoms.
2. Physicians and practitioners would rather refer to a rheumatologist than diagnose or manage arthritis patients.
3. Unfortunately, the impediments to such care are numerous. Instead of referral rules, referring doctors and patients would rather have easy access.
4. There will be 75,000 new RA patients in the USA every year, but to capture these, rheumatologists must see many more, as less than 10% of new referrals will have RA.
5. The best way to attract a new RA patient is for rheumatologists to modify their consultative intake processes to accommodate the growing number of patients with musculoskeletal symptoms, some of whom will have early RA.

So what is happening now? A total of 446 U.S. rheumatologists surveyed in 2008 reported seeing 15.4 patients per day in an average 4-day work week and spending 21.7 min with follow-up patients and 50 min with each new patient consultation [5]. On average, they see 5.5 RA follow-up patients and about 1 new inflammatory arthritis patient per day. These numbers underscore why rheumatologists don't see more patients with early disease; their scheduling processes won't allow it. The approach for new and follow-up patients is essentially the same, with more time afforded new patients for more data gathering. The current work processes slow down the rheumatologist at a time when rapid assessments and decision-making should be in effect. In 2011, 605 rheumatologists were asked, "Who should evaluate patients with undiagnosed joint, muscle, or widespread pains?" 57% thought this responsibility should rest with the PCP, but 82% felt rheumatologists were most effective in doing it! This reflects a broken system in which those physicians who most often see these patients have not been prepared to provide effective evaluations, and those who are most skilled at such evaluations are not practicing in ways that allow them to do the greatest good for the largest number of patients that require their services.

My studies also found that the rheumatologists who see a high number of early inflammatory arthritis patients are those with wait times under 2 weeks. These large group practices or innovative individuals have found ways to expedite new patient consults. As the number of rheumatologists is predicted to decline in the next 10 years, according to the American College of Rheumatology's 2007 manpower survey [6], the rising need for rheumatology consultative services can only be accomplished by limiting the rheumatologist's initial visit to diagnosing the problem and setting up later evaluations and treatments as needed. Some studies also suggest that highly trained clinical nurse specialists can provide more accurate initial screening for musculoskeletal symptoms than less prepared PCPs who are faced with the entire spectrum of human illnesses.

Skilled diagnosticians can utilize pattern recognition, expertise, and clinical skills to derive an accurate diagnosis or an efficient plan for further evaluation, while seeing more new patients in fewer minutes. Such a transformation does not require more rheumatologists or physician extenders, it only requires rheumatologists to work smarter, not harder. This can be accomplished with a change in scheduling patterns, a focus on high yield evaluation processes, and confidence in one's diagnostic acumen.

Eric Newman, the coeditor of this book, and his colleagues at the Geisinger Medical Center achieved this by developing an "open access" approach for all new referral appointments [7]. Developing a process that guarantees same day or same week appointments ensures the earliest possible evaluation of those in need. The key elements included dedication to change and the requirement to study and modify their scheduling processes using continuous process improvement methods. The net result of their transformation was increased intake volume, more early RA patients, greater patient satisfaction, dramatically reduced wait times, and greater productivity and higher income.

Measuring Up

Measuring disease activity is central to the effective management of RA and many other chronic diseases. The results define the need for treatment, and for adjusting it, to achieve and maintain control. There is no single piece of clinical information or lab test that provides this for RA. Multiple pieces of data must be collected and analyzed. Not only does active RA reflect itself in multiple ways, but other conditions may produce similar "masquerader" symptoms.

Rheumatologists have traditionally judged the patient's progress and response to therapy by "gestalt," a subjective assessment based on whatever clinical information they happen to collect through questioning, examination, and review of tests and X-rays. This information not only varies from visit to visit, but widely among rheumatologists. The gestalt approach contrasts with standardized quantitative clinical measurements that are used to measure RA disease activity in clinical drug trials, and are currently derived from seven core set variables. These are either numbers or estimates reported on visual analog scales, or questionnaires: tender joint count (TJC), swollen joint count (SJC), the physician global assessment of the patient's disease activity, the patient global assessment, patient-reported pain, lab tests for inflammation (the sedimentation rate or C-reactive protein), and a standardized patient report of functional disability, such as the Health Assessment Questionnaire. Visual analog scales are ten-point lines on which the physician or patient makes a mark to represent the severity from low to high pain or controlled to high disease activity, as examples.

Drs. Fredrick Wolfe and Theodore Pincus, two leading academic rheumatologists, took clinical measurement of RA disease activity to the next level by validating the importance of symptoms and functional status reported by patients on standardized questionnaires, referred to as patient-reported outcome measures (PROMs). PROMs have become important in both clinical trials and daily patient care, outperforming traditional joint counts, tests for inflammation, or joint erosions on X-rays in predicting disability, functional decline, need for joint replacement surgery, and death [8]. Moreover, what the patient reports on a standardized questionnaire, such as Dr. Pincus' RAPID form, is available to the physician without any investment of additional time for questioning. But many rheumatologists continue to prefer what they observe personally in developing their "gestalt" disease activity assessment.

Combinations of clinical information known as composite scores have been used increasingly to standardize disease activity measurement in trials and practice. For example, the calculated disease activity score (DAS) was developed in Europe to dynamically define disease activity level and drug response, as were the American College of Rheumatology (ACR) response measures in the US to distinguish drug responses from placebo responses in trials of new drugs [9, 10]. While these composite measures have invigorated drug development, they are impractical in the routine outpatient clinic where time limits data gathering, lab measures may not be available at the time of service, and the complexity of the DAS and ACR calculations impede real-time treatment planning. So these initial composite measures did not replace the gestalt for routine care.

Professor Joseph Smolen of Vienna and colleagues have since developed more practical composite measures specifically for clinical practice, such as the Clinical Disease Activity Index (CDAI) (the sum of the Physician's and Patient's Global Assessments of Disease Activity + the Tender and Swollen Joint Counts). They validated the CDAI against the gold standard DAS [11, 12]. In my own clinics, I developed a one-page patient evaluation form that includes a patient pain score,

Table 15.2 Various composite disease activity measures for clinical trials and patient care include a variety of clinical data elements

	Patient function	Patient pain	Patient global	Physician global	Tender joint count	Swollen joint count	Lab tests
ACR20	X	X	X	X	X	X	ESR CRP
DAS28			X	X	X	X	ESR
SDAI			X	X	X	X	CRP
CDAI			X	X	X	X	
GAS	X	X			X		

All of these reflect disease activity, but composite measures that can be calculated during patient evaluations provide greater value in guiding treatment than those that require laboratory data or complex calculations

ACR20 American College of Rheumatology 20% response, *DAS28* Disease Activity Score 28 joint count, *SDAI* Simplified Disease Activity Index, *CDAI* Clinical Disease Activity Index, *GAS* Global Arthritis Score, *ESR* Erythrocyte Sedimentation Rate, *CRP* C-Reactive Protein (inflammation tests)

Fig. 15.1 Correlation of the Global Arthritis Score (GAS) and DAS28 scores in 64 RA patients (244 visits) seen in an outpatient clinic (Spearman Rank Correlation, $R = 0.88$). Values for the two composite measures show a high degree of agreement

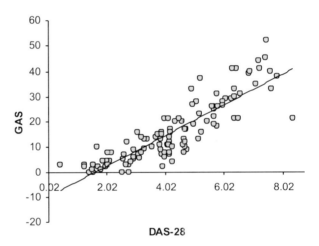

a patient global assessment, their indication of which joints are painful on a diagram, and a check list of common daily activities. This facilitates standardized data collection, disease activity measurement, and electronic record use. (Appendix A) It became the basis for calculating the Global Arthritis Score (GAS) (the sum of the patient's pain and functional assessment scores, and the number of tender joints) [13]. The patient completes the form in the waiting room, and GAS is calculated by the nurse as a vital sign before the physician begins their evaluation.

The components of several commonly used composite scores are shown in Table 15.2. While they differ somewhat in their specific components, they correlate highly with one another (Fig. 15.1) and provide similarly valuable information. Their use has grown significantly, but is still uncommon. My last survey of 446 US rheumatologists in 2008 showed that only 12% were using the DAS in practice, and fewer still were using other alternatives: the RAPID3 (3%), CDAI (2%), GAS (2%), and SDAI (1%) [5]. It is not as important which measure a rheumatologist uses, as whether she/he uses one of the alternatives.

Two important questions are

1. Why should these disease activity measures be used in practice?, and
2. Why are so few rheumatologists using them?

The first answer is easy: these practice-friendly disease activity measures have been shown repeatedly to outperform "routine care" using gestalt. These benefits were shown convincingly in the "TICORA" (tight control of RA) study several years ago. Grigor and colleagues studied 110 RA patients with less than 5 years of RA [14]. Half received routine care by their rheumatologist every 3 months, and the other half were managed intensively with monthly visits and DAS28 measurements. Treatment was accelerated in the "intensive" group at a minimum of every 3 months until a DAS under 2.4 was achieved, indicating that the patient's disease was in remission. After 18 months, the treat to target (T2T) group was receiving higher doses of single DMARDs and more combination drug treatments (67 vs. 11% of control patients), and they had experienced a fourfold higher rate of measurable remission (65 versus 16%). Several other trials have shown similar outcomes employing metric-driven management strategies [15, 16].

Answering the second question, "Why are measures not being used widely?" is more complex. To begin, physicians tend to overestimate the results of treatment in the absence of using precise measurements. A famous quote from Dr. Verna Wright states, "Clinicians may all too easily spend years writing "doing well" in the notes of a patient who has become progressively crippled before their eyes" [17]. Again from my 2008 survey, 446 US rheumatologists claimed to achieve remission for 32% of their RA patients [5]. This is surprising for several reasons:

1. The same survey showed that the vast majority of these rheumatologists do not use standardized measurements, so how do they know?
2. Other studies show that even when using highly effective biologic drugs, rheumatologists practicing routinely achieve remissions in less than 35–45% of their RA patients [17, 18].
3. Patients in practice do not achieve the same level of clinical responses achieved in randomized controlled clinical trials [19].
4. Rheumatologists are slow to change DMARD therapies in the face of moderate-to-severe disease activity [20–22].

Metric-dependent decision-making relies instead on well-defined numeric benchmarks for remission, and low, moderate, and high disease activity. In my clinic, the GAS is used to assess disease activity and to gauge the patient's progress toward achieving remission, the goal being a GAS <3.

There are several other reasons, all unfounded or ill-advised, for rheumatologists failing to use metrics in practice, including (1) the belief that measuring outcomes takes time – studies show it only takes 90 s to do a 28 joint count and under 20 s to calculate the GAS or RAPID3 [23]; (2) such measures are not taught in most rheumatology training programs, although this is slowly changing; and (3) metrics are not required for being paid, although the Medicare pay-for-performance program will require and reward metrics use in practice.

My own experience has taught me several clear lessons. First, the GAS can be easily incorporated into all rheumatology visits. Each patient's report of their pain level, function, and TJC is useful in their care whether they have RA or one of the other common rheumatic diseases – osteoarthritis, gout, polymyalgia rheumatica, fibromyalgia, psoriatic arthritis, etc. Second, the GAS measure generally agrees with one's gestalt; however, its value-added is apparent in up to 15% of RA patients where it leads to earlier and more effective treatment. Lastly, measuring isn't a goal unto itself, but a reflection of a commitment to excellence. Hence, one must measure and treat to a measurable target goal to arrive at an optimal outcome for the patient.

Treat to Target

T2T care aims to control RA by rapidly accelerating drug therapy in response to a measure showing active disease until sustained control is documented [24]. T2T's pillars are early treatment and validated measurement of disease activity – the principles I reviewed already. Growing numbers of studies support this approach in comparison to "regular" care [14, 24–28], and these have now been combined into confirmatory meta-analyses as well [27, 28]. TICORA was first, as described in the prior section. Another, the BeST study, confirmed TICORA and went on to show that the T2T patients had less joint damage after 2–4 years, even though the "regular" care patients eventually achieved similar disease control through more gradual treatment acceleration – RA damages joints early on. We still need to learn whether T2T reduces joint damage and preserves patients' function across the years, and whether the higher short-term costs of more intensive treatment pay off in longer-term cost reductions, less disability, and survival advantages.

Tight control is the key to managing most chronic disorders such as diabetes, hypertension, and asthma, yet it remains a challenge for most rheumatologists treating RA. While many believe they are providing tight control, few employ metrics, so they can't actually recognize that they are undertreating. Even fewer quicken therapy dependably, whether they are measuring or not. Rheumatologists, like other physicians, change slowly, but a growing number are opting for using the DAS, CDAI, RAPID3 or GAS, and for T2T management. Pay-for-performance and other reimbursement changes in the US will support measurement and T2T becoming the standard of care and will provide greater patient comfort and satisfaction.

Personalized Medicine for RA

As the effective treatment options for RA have increased over the last 30 years, it has become clear that different patients respond differently, and not surprisingly, because individual patients' RA varies – not only their drug responses, but onset when young or old, small or large joints involved, RA blood test negative or positive. Our best evidence-based therapies are effective in less than half of patients, and fewer than 10% will go into remission on any single treatment. Presently, we determine best treatments for individuals by trying single drugs and combinations until the best response is obtained. Worse is our inability to predict who will develop adverse effects: methotrexate liver injury, anti-malarial eye injury, or vertebral compression fractures from steroid treatment.

We need to become still better at choosing treatments for individuals, and personalized medicine offers this promise. This refers to tailoring health care to the individual guided by their genetic, metabolic, and nutritional testing profiles. The human genome project and advances in biotechnology and biostatistics are enabling such complex testing and analyses. Personalized medicine research is drawing great interest and greater dollars from philanthropists, venture capitalists, mega-millionaires like Mark Cuban (owner of Dallas Mavericks and HDnet), the pharmaceutical industry, the FDA, the NIH, and leading medical institutions like Stanford University, the Cleveland Clinic, and Baylor Research Institute, to name a few.

At the Baylor Research Institute, we are exploring how biomarkers of inflammation and genomic identifiers in RA patients relate to their individual drug responsiveness and toxicity susceptibilities. We have begun using genotyping to guide treatment for difficult to control RA patients. As one example, a woman who had failed many commonly used treatments over 6 years has now been in remission for 18 months on a rarely used biologic drug (anakinra) that was suggested by her genotyping. As the number of specifically targeted biological drugs for RA increases, our goal is to use testing rather than trial-and-error to identify the best choices for individual patients from the outset. Personalized medicine aspires to rapid treatment, remissions, and dramatic alterations in disease course with high-yield, low-risk therapies.

Improving Healthcare Outcomes in Rheumatoid Arthritis (Table 15.3)

> *The major obstacles to change are routine behavior and the belief that change is difficult. The baseball movie "League of Their Own" is famous for the quote, "There's no crying in baseball." from manager Jimmie Dugan, played by Tom Hanks. His other great quote, was, "It's supposed to be hard... being hard is what makes it great. If it weren't hard everyone would do it."*
>
>   John J. Cush

I believe each of these priorities represents a highly important change in the delivery of healthcare to patients with RA. Rheumatologists need to adopt them; patients need to insist on them; and payers must begin to demand them. Each is rooted in improving disease outcomes, patients' quality of life, and long-term costs of care. While most rheumatologists believe the next great advances in RA care will depend on new drug discovery and development, I believe that changes in practice routines and performance will be more critical. Whereas new drugs will more effectively control symptoms and disease activity, changes in practice processes

Table 15.3 Priorities in RA care

New RA treatment rules	"The bottom line"
1. Diagnose and treat early	Reduce wait times and create access by improving practice processes
2. Measure disease activity	Use composite disease activity measures routinely on all patients
3. Treat to Target (T2T): Use the best drug first; More combinations and biologics	Based on active disease and the presence of poor prognostic factors. (The data show that RA is undertreated)
4. Provide personalized care	Using practice metrics and Treating to Target yields a four times ↑ in remissions
5. Avoid toxicity	Rather than respond to adverse events, it's best to avoid toxicity through careful patient selection, tailored screening, and monitoring according to the treatment chosen
6. Identify and treat other conditions that accompany RA (comorbidities)	Manage the "whole patient" cooperatively by the PCP and rheumatologist

will provide these benefits in a more timely and accurate manner, increasing the odds of disease control or remission. We can do much more with what we have available now and will have in the future.

Editor's Comment. Addressing the care gaps in access, measurement, and treatment are repeating themes across chronic diseases and the improvement stories told by our authors. Jack Cush has defined and tested opportunities for closing these gaps in rheumatoid arthritis care that are not only informing his rheumatology colleagues, but can help others, and benefit patients. His use of e-mail questionnaires to assess the status of care in rheumatology practices is novel, and helpful in creating performance expectations. JTH

References

1. McKay C, Veinot P, Badley EM. Characteristics of evolving models of care for arthritis: a key informant study. BMC Health Serv Res. 2008;8:147.
2. Maradit-Kremers H et al. Increased unrecognized coronary heart disease and sudden deaths in rheumatoid arthritis: a population-based cohort study. Arthritis Rheum. 2005;52:402–11.
3. Cush JJ, Weinblatt ME, Kavanaugh A. Rheumatoid arthritis: Early diagnosis and treatment. Cush JJ, Weinblatt ME, Kavanaugh A, editors. Professional communications, 2nd edn, New York, 2007.
4. Cush JJ. Remodeling the rheumatology practice to facilitate early referral. Rheum Dis Clin North Am. 2005;31:591–604.
5. Cush JJ. Trends in US Rheumatology practice: a survey of US rheumatologists. Arthritis Rheum. 2008;58(Suppl):S747.
6. Deal C et al. The United States rheumatology workforce: supply and demand, 2005–2025. Arthritis Rheum. 2007;56:722–9.
7. Newman ED, Harrington TM, Olenginski TP, Perruquet JL, McKinley K. "The rheumatologist can see you now": Successful implementation of an advanced access model in a rheumatology practice. Arthritis Rheum. 2004;51:253–7.

8. Pincus T, Callahan LF, Brooks RH, Fuchs HA, Olsen NJ, Kaye JJ. Self-report questionnaire scores in rheumatoid arthritis compared with traditional physical, radiographic, and laboratory measures. Ann Int Med. 1989;110:259–66.
9. van der Heijde DM, van't Hof MA, van Riel PL. Disease activity score. Ann Rheum Dis. 1992; 51:140.
10. Felson DT, Anderson JJ, Boers M, Bombardier C, Chernoff M, Fried B, et al. The American College of Rheumatology preliminary core set of disease activity measures for rheumatoid arthritis clinical trials. The Committee on Outcome Measures in Rheumatoid Arthritis Clinical Trials. Arthritis Rheum. 1993;36:729–40.
11. Smolen JS, Breedveld BF, Schiff MH, Kalden JR, Emery P, Eberl G, et al. A simplified disease activity index for rheumatoid arthritis for use in clinical practice. Rheumatology. 2003;42:244–57.
12. Aletaha D, Nell VPK, Stamm T, Uffmann M, Pflugbell S, Machold K, et al. Acute phase reactants add little to composite disease activity indices for rheumatoid arthritis: validation of a clinical activity score. Ann Rheum Dis. 2005;64 Suppl 3:209.
13. Cush JJ. Global arthritis score: a rapid practice tool for rheumatoid arthritis (RA) assessment. Arthritis Rheum. 2005;52(Suppl):S686.
14. Grigor C, Capell H, Stirling A, McMahon AD, Lock P, Vallance R, et al. Effect of a treatment strategy of tight control for rheumatoid arthritis (the TICORA study): a single-blind randomised controlled trial. Lancet. 2004;364:263–9.
15. Verstappen SM, Jacobs JW, van der Veen MJ, Heurkens AH, Schenk Y, ter Borg EJ, et al. Utrecht Rheumatoid Arthritis Cohort study group. Intensive treatment with methotrexate in early rheumatoid arthritis: aiming for remission. Computer Assisted Management in Early Rheumatoid Arthritis (CAMERA, an open-label strategy trial). Ann Rheum Dis. 2007;66:1443–9.
16. Fransen J, Moens HB, Speyer I, van Riel PL. Effectiveness of systematic monitoring of rheumatoid arthritis disease activity in daily practice: a multicentre, cluster randomised controlled trial. Ann Rheum Dis. 2005;64(9):1294–8.
17. Gibofsky A, Palmar WR, Goldman JA, et al. Real-world utilization of DMARDs and biologics in rheumatoid arthritis: the RADIUS (Rheumatoid Arthritis Disease-modifying Anti-rheumatic Drug intervention and Utilization Study) study. Curr Med Res Opin. 2006;22(1):169–83.
18. Weissman MH, et al. Analysis at 2 years of an inception cohort of early rheumatoid arthritis: The SONORA Study. EULAR 2004; Abstract OP0042.
19. Kievit W, Fransen J, Oerlemans AJ, Kuper HH, van der Laar MA, de Rooij DJ, et al. The efficacy of anti-TNF in rheumatoid arthritis, a comparison between randomised controlled trials and clinical practice. Ann Rheum Dis. 2007;66:1473–8.
20. Harrison MJ et al. Arthritis Rheum. 2005;52(9 suppl):S720.
21. Kahn KL et al. Application of explicit process of care measurement to rheumatoid arthritis: moving from evidence to practice. Arthritis Rheum. 2006;55:884–91.
22. Saraux A et al. Most rheumatologists are conservative in active rheumatoid arthritis despite methotrexate therapy: results of the PRISME survey. J Rheumatol. 2006;33(7):1258–65.
23. Yazici Y et al. Time to score quantitative rheumatoid arthritis measures: 28-Joint Count, Disease Activity Score, Health Assessment Questionnaire (HAQ), Multidimensional HAQ (MDHAQ), and Routine Assessment of Patient Index Data (RAPID) scores. J Rheumatol. 2008;35:603–9.
24. Smolen JS et al. Treating rheumatoid arthritis to target: recommendations of an international task force. Ann Rheum Dis. 2010;69(4):631–7.
25. Goekoop-Ruiterman YPM et al. Clinical and radiographic outcomes of four different treatment strategies in patients with early rheumatoid arthritis (the BeSt study): a randomized, controlled trial. Arthritis Rheum. 2005;52:3381–90.
26. Van der Kooij SM et al. Clinical and radiological efficacy of initial vs delayed treatment with infliximab plus methotrexate in patients with early rheumatoid arthritis. Ann Rheum Dis. 2009;68:1153–8.
27. Schoels M et al. Evidence for treating rheumatoid arthritis to target: results of a systematic literature search. Ann Rheum Dis. 2010;69(4):638–43.
28. Schipper LG, van Hulst LT, Grol R, van Riel PL, Hulscher ME, Fransen J. Meta-analysis of tight control strategies in rheumatoid arthritis: protocolized treatment has additional value with respect to the clinical outcome. Rheumatology (Oxford). 2010;49(11):2154–64.

Chapter 16
Heart Failure: Reducing Readmissions

Kathi Farrell and Kathleen Sullivan

Keywords Heart failure • Marian Medical Center • Program coordinator • Chronic disease • Readmission • Disease management program • Monitoring

Heart failure, often known as congestive heart failure (CHF), occurs when the heart cannot pump enough blood and oxygen to support other organs. The term heart failure is often used incorrectly to describe other cardiac conditions such as myocardial infarction (heart attack) or cardiac arrest. This is a serious condition, but one which responds well to certain medications, clinical oversight, and life style changes.

About 5.8 million people in the United States have heart failure. About 670,000 people are diagnosed with it each year [1]. According to the American Heart Association Statistics Committee and Stroke Statistics Subcommittee:

- About one in five people who have heart failure die within 1 year from diagnosis.
- Heart failure was a contributing cause of 282,754 deaths in 2006.
- In 2010, heart failure will cost the United States $39.2 billion. This total includes the cost of healthcare services, medications, and lost productivity.
- The most common causes of heart failure are coronary artery disease, high blood pressure, and diabetes.
- Early diagnosis and treatment can improve quality of life as well as life expectancy for people who have heart failure. Treatment usually involves taking medication, reducing salt in the diet, getting daily physical activity, and the careful management of any symptoms that may develop.

K. Farrell, RN, BSN, PHN (✉) • K. Sullivan, RN, MSN
Marian Medical Center, Catholic HealthCare West, Santa Maria, CA, USA
e-mail: kathi.farrell@chw.edu

J.T. Harrington and E.D. Newman (eds.), *Great Health Care: Making It Happen*,   137
DOI 10.1007/978-1-4614-1198-7_16, © Springer Science+Business Media, LLC 2012

Heart Failure and Hospitalization

Heart failure is a disabling, potentially deadly, and costly condition. It causes a decrease in both physical and mental health, including depression as is common with all chronic diseases. It worsens with time, with the exception of correctable causes such as heart valve disorders.

Each year approximately 27% of patients on Medicare diagnosed with heart failure during a hospitalization are readmitted within 30 days of discharge. Such unplanned readmissions cost Medicare $17.4 billion a year, and heart failure is the most frequent reason for rehospitalizations [2]. Disease management programs can dramatically improve readmission rates, the cost of care, and the quality of life for those living with this disease.

Patients with heart failure also have a high incidence of comorbidities, such as chronic obstructive pulmonary disease, dementia, renal failure, hypertension, and diabetes. Comorbid conditions greatly influence the rate of rehospitalization for patients with heart failure, and need to be included in planning for the post-acute care needs of any person discharged with heart failure.

The Institute for Healthcare Improvement, along with the Robert Wood Johnson (RWJ) Foundation, outlined an ideal transition-to-the-home environment for patients with heart failure that has reduced 30-day readmission rates from 15 to 6% [3]. Their recommendations included the following:

- Enhanced admissions assessment – Standardized care assessment should identify all needs postdischarge, and discharge planning that addresses these needs.
- Enhanced teaching and learning – Patient and family education should include verbal as well as written instructions, identifying barriers to understanding and reinforcement of education.
- Patient- and family-centered handoff communication – Focusing on discharge from the time of admission allows patients and caregivers to understand the care plan that will be followed on discharge. This should include medication reconciliation: addressing any discrepancies in medication, ensuring availability of medications on discharge, as well as any community resources that may be necessary.
- Postdischarge acute care – Postdischarge acute follow-up care within 48 h should be addressed prior to discharge for high-risk patients (those who have been admitted twice in 1 year with heart failure), and patients with barriers to learning. Home health is often a bridge between the hospital and any disease management program and/or follow up with a physician.

Marian Medical Center (MMC) CHF Program (Fig. 16.1)

MMC's chronic disease management program for CHF was originally envisioned by, and partially funded through the RWJ Foundation as a leadership project while one of us (Kathleen Sullivan) was an RWJ Executive Nurse Fellow. We have

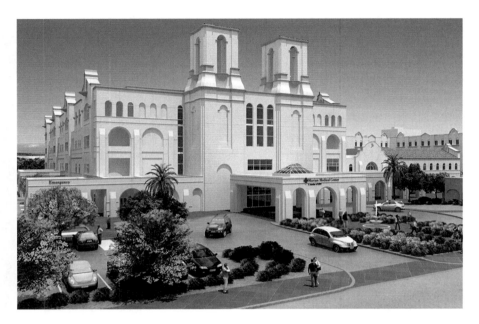

Fig. 16.1 Marian Medical Center, Santa Maria, CA

followed over 1,000 patients since its inception in 2002. In 2008, the program was replicated in two other hospitals in our service area.

The literature shows that the majority of programs such as ours do not exceed 6 months duration of care. Since we were seeing less than 1% readmissions for our patients at 1 year, we reduced the enrollment period to 6 months as well in 2008, and we focused our interactions on the first 30 days after discharge. If patients are not readmitted and/or seen in the ER for a heart failure exacerbation within 6 months, we discharge them. Patients know they can call us at any time with any questions, requests for resources, etc. If a patient is readmitted with a diagnosis of CHF, we reopen their file and begin the process again. We have monitored the effects of this change, and have not seen any negative impacts on our clinical outcomes to date. This change did, however, decrease our average census in F/Y 2009. As this program is provided regardless of payer or other contractual obligations, this change has conserved resources.

Initially, we required a physician referral to the program. Most often, this was received while the patient was already hospitalized. In February 2010, the Medical Executive Committee reviewed the results of this outpatient program, and unanimously decided that all CHF patients should be enrolled without requiring a physician order. This recent change has afforded our nurse clinicians more timely access to all heart failure patients, and has improved our capacity to track them and provide real-time services from the outset.

This policy change is responsible for an increase in clients enrolled/fiscal year:

- In 2007, 164 new clients were enrolled = average census 124
- In 2008, 150 new clients were enrolled = average census 122

- In 2009, 175 new clients were enrolled = average census of 97
- In 2010, 236 new clients were enrolled = average census of 110

The CHF Program Coordinator now receives notice upon admission or an ER visit for all CHF patients, and attempts to see them right away. She provides education mandated by The Joint Commission regarding heart failure diagnosis, exacerbation of heart failure, the importance of daily weights, low sodium diets, medication compliance, and appropriate follow up with physicians. The outpatient program is explained to patients at the same time.

Self-care is notoriously poor in persons with heart failure, despite concentrated efforts by nurses to educate them about how to care for themselves. Surprisingly, about 25% of the clients eligible for the CHF Program refuse it; participation is voluntary. Networking with similar disease management programs reveals that this is not unique. Assisting patients in skill development requires a shift in the patient education module from traditional authoritarian approach to patient-centered, collaborative education [4]. We ask simple, open-ended questions, provide information regarding diets, weight monitoring, and exacerbation of symptoms, and follow up by mailing literature to support our discussions.

Marian's Heart Failure Program utilizes the following evidence-based strategies to educate patients and manage the care, consistent with other programs described in the literature:

- Education about Heart Failure including

  - Signs and symptoms of exacerbation/what to look for and report
  - Information regarding low sodium diets
  - The importance of daily weights

- Fluid restriction (if indicated)
- Medication instructions and compliance
- Activity level
- Follow-up appointments
- Information regarding any other comorbidities and their effect on the management of heart failure.

Regular follow-up calls are then scheduled for 6 months to assess patient compliance and understanding. Our basic postdischarge algorithm is to follow a patient weekly for 1 month, every other week for 2 months, and then monthly for a total of 6 months, although the frequency of follow up can be customized to meet the patient's needs. Our program is predominantly telephonic, although we do schedule meetings with clients when necessary. The program coordinator serves as a partner to the physician and other members of the healthcare team, and as a liaison and advocate for and between the patient and the healthcare team.

Over the years, we have consistently experienced readmission rates of less than 1% within 30 days for patients with a diagnosis of CHF enrolled in our management program. This is a critical time point from both a quality and cost perspective, as avoiding readmissions is key to hospitals succeeding in today's healthcare environment. Of clients readmitted to MMC within 30 days, however, 45% expired or were discharged to Hospice, indicating the high mortality associated with readmissions. We now measure our readmission rates for CHF within 6 months as well, and again, the result is less than 1%.

In 2010, we experienced an unusually high number of readmissions compared to other years, and this group also demonstrated the high mortality associated with read-mission of CHF patients. Fifty patients accounted for 55 total readmissions to MMC within 31 days of discharge in 2010, 47% with a primary CHF diagnosis. One expired within a month, a second expired within 6 weeks, and 45% have expired since or are currently on Hospice service. Only two of these patients had consented to participate in the CHF Program after their initial hospitalization for a variety of reasons.

Our program started with one full-time RN Coordinator. A part-time bilingual nurse was added in 2007. She spends 4 h/week at two community clinics within our delivery system that serve a predominantly Spanish-speaking population, and the same number at the local public health department. Her networking with providers and scheduling appointments with clients increased our underserved population from 41% of the total enrolled to 48% in the last fiscal year.

We believe the extraordinary efforts of our program coordinators are key to our clients' well-being and our unusually low readmission rate. These include work with the patient and the family to procure necessary community resources, and their collaboration with other MMS disease management program colleagues. Medications are obtained at no/low cost, meals at home are arranged for our home-bound clients, and orders are requested from providers when needed for home health nursing ser-vices, physical therapy, a medical social worker, or Hospice at the end of life. We also provide information regarding Advance Care Directives, and are able to enroll our clients in our Osteoporosis and Diabetes self-management training programs, and to consult the Palliative Care team. This system flexibility and collaboration provides chronic disease management seamlessly to many of our patients, including those with multiple comorbidities.

Currently, we use an electronic disease management program that includes initial follow up and medication assessments. We are developing advanced clinical mod-ules for our program as part of a system-wide electronic health record transition.

A Patient Success Story

He lived alone with no local relatives when he was seen for an initial assessment by our CHF Program coordinator after an ER visit. At the end of the interview, he readily agreed to have information mailed to him. When the nurse contacted him the following week, he admitted he was legally blind and unable to read the material. This had not been reported anywhere in his history and physical or dis-charge summary. The nurse contacted a local volunteer agency to arrange for someone to visit him on a weekly basis. His phone was programmed to contact his physician, pharmacy, emergency services, and our office; the font size of all mailed information was increased so he could read it with his magnifying glass, and a volunteer was arranged to read to him as well. A "talking scale" was also obtained to assist with food measurement. Community resource providers not only became new friends, but his health improved, and he required no further ER visits or hospitalizations.

The Future

We have been very pleased with the success of our telephonic care management program thus far, but are enthusiastic about adding additional components to further improve service to these medically fragile patients, enhance our capacity to manage more patients with our limited resources, and continue improving our readmission rate. The rollout of a robust electronic health record will expand our disease management, documentation, and communications with other system providers. We are piloting a remote patient monitoring system for weight, vital signs, symptoms, medication compliance, and disease state knowledge. These in-home monitors will transmit clinical data real-time to the care coordinator to enable more timely interventions. We will assess whether they prevent hospitalizations. We intend next to add physician-approved medical protocols including medication titration parameters (e.g., furosemide) that the RN can utilize when symptom exacerbations threaten ER visits or hospitalization. These additions to our already successful program will enable us to provide cutting-edge disease management support to the patients we serve.

Editor's comments: I was invited to visit Marian Medical Center in bucolic Santa Maria, California several years ago by Dr. Mary Otes to assist in developing their osteoporosis management program. She introduced me to Kathi Farrell who was already doing everything for their heart failure population that I was suggesting for osteoporosis care. My advice to Mary, "Do for your hip fracture patients what Kathi is doing, and coordinate the programs across diseases." And now they are. The Marian experience demonstrates the value of nurse management supported by disease population registries. Their performance monitoring and continuous improvement approach are exemplary. In addition, MMC is a smaller community hospital within a larger, highly effective hospital network, and is on the same page with its independent medical staff. JTH

References

1. Lloyd-Jones D, Adams RJ, Brown TM, et al. Heart disease and stroke statistics – 2010 update. A report from the American Heart Association. Circulation. 2010;121:e46–215.
2. Jencks SF, Williams MV, Coleman EA. Rehospitalizations among patients in the Medicare fee-for-service program. N Engl J Med. 2009;360(14):1418–28.
3. Nielsen GA, et al. Transforming care at the bedside how-to guide: creating an ideal transition home for patients with heart failure. Institute for Healthcare Improvement. www.ihi.org. Accessed 16 Feb 2010.
4. Dickson V, Riegel B. Are we teaching what patients need to know? Building skills in heart failure self-care. Heart Lung. 2009;38:253–61.

Chapter 17
Chronic Kidney Disease: Changing the Mean by Changing the *Mien*

Jerry Yee, Mark D. Faber, and Sandeep S. Soman

Keywords Chronic kidney disease • Mien • Henry Ford Hospital • CKD • ESRD • System-based CKD care • DMAIC • Database • CPOE

Mien: Bearing or manner, especially as it reveals an inner state of mind.

What follows is a description of how our group of nephrologists transformed the delivery of healthcare to our patient population with chronic kidney disease (CKD) over 8 years. This required significant changes in our mindset and attitudes. The changes primarily involved adopting a highly automated and protocol-driven style of care that was geared toward efficiency without a sacrifice in quality. Our emphasis was delivery of high quality, relevant, evidence-based, patient-centered, multidisciplinary care with enthusiastic and dedicated participation by a broad coalition of involved stakeholders, not only nephrologists, but also internal medicine trainees and faculty, family medicine physicians, the clinical laboratory staff, nurse practitioners, social workers, pharmacists, and dietitians.

The Challenge of Chronic Kidney Disease at Henry Ford Hospital

The Henry Ford Hospital is the flagship of the Henry Ford Health System and is located within the City of Detroit. It is an 802-bed urban, tertiary care institution that serves a large contingent of the Detroit medical population. Patients with end-stage renal disease (ESRD) can receive all modalities of renal replacement therapy within Henry Ford, which includes a wholly owned dialysis organization.

J. Yee, MD (✉) • M D. Faber • S.S. Soman, MD
Division of Nephrology, Henry Ford Hospital, Detroit, MI, USA
e-mail: jyee1@hfhs.org

J.T. Harrington and E.D. Newman (eds.), *Great Health Care: Making It Happen*,
DOI 10.1007/978-1-4614-1198-7_17, © Springer Science+Business Media, LLC 2012

Nearly 82% of Detroit residents are African American, according to the United States Census 2000, a population recognized to be at high risk for CKD [1]. Detroit has the dubious distinction of being the most obese city in the United States [2], and greater frequencies of hypertension, obesity, and diabetes contribute disproportionally to CKD risk. In fact, data from the United States Renal Data Survey reported that Detroit had one of the highest prevalences of ESRD from 1996 to 2006 [3]. These realities convinced us that a *tsunami* of CKD and ESRD was converging on our healthcare system, and that these patients would overwhelm our already substantial ESRD provider system. A mathematically irrefutable truth emerged: CKD progression to ESRD would have to be slowed to maintain the equilibrium between patients entering and exiting our ESRD portals, and this slowing would have to be accomplished in the nondialysis-dependent, earlier stage CKD population.

Many of our patients had first presented with advanced stage CKD prior to our early efforts to change in 2002. They seldom understood their illness and its complications, even as they initiated dialysis. For years, the National Kidney Foundation of Michigan had been developing and implementing strategies and projects that improved the lives of kidney allograft recipients and those requiring other renal replacement therapies. However, strategies to identify persons with earlier stage CKD and to forestall its progression were lacking. The National Kidney Foundation's free Kidney Early Evaluation Program (KEEP) was implemented in Detroit to assist in the earlier detection of CKD, but these results would not be available for several years [4]. In addition, because our healthcare system was not chosen as the Detroit KEEP site, we could not easily participate in this early recognition exercise. Therefore, we would have to gather our own data and act upon it.

Our group attacked the problem of CKD in metropolitan Detroit, and specifically within our healthcare system, through a combined approach of dedicated and widespread educational efforts, implementing the Modification of Diet in Renal Disease estimated glomerular filtration rate (eGFR) equation, and fundamentally changing how we approached, identified, diagnosed, and treated CKD [5]. We were determined to ameliorate the impending and largely unrecognized CKD crisis with an expected prevalence of 13% in U.S. adults and an even higher prevalence in our own patients [6].

A Two-Pronged Strategy for System-Based CKD Care

We planned two major and parallel strategies: (a) redesigning and renaming our renal disease clinic as a CKD Clinic and (b) partnering with local healthcare groups and the National Kidney Foundation of Michigan to implement global strategies for reducing the "big three" risk factors for CKD – obesity, hypertension, and diabetes. Furthermore, we recognized another "big three" of comorbid diseases that represent a formidable challenge for primary care physicians (PCPs), nephrologists, cardiologists, endocrinologists, and affected patients – diabetes; cardiovascular disease manifested as angina, myocardial infarction, and heart failure; and CKD [7].

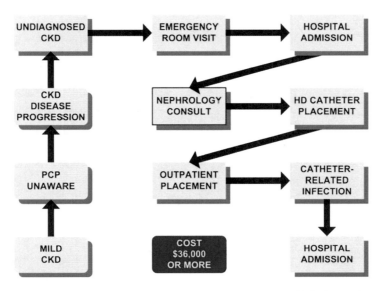

Fig. 17.1 Suboptimal progression pathway of chronic kidney disease (CKD) into end-stage renal disease relates to underrecognition of CKD, with consequent hospitalization and hemodialysis (HD) catheter placement for urgent hemodialysis that may be complicated by catheter-related infection and repetitive hospitalization. Healthcare system costs amount to approximately $36,000 USD or more when this pathway is followed

Effective management of these patients warrants exquisite, multidisciplinary collaborations that include nephrologists [8]. With successful management, the pernicious pathway trod by half of our ESRD patients could be averted.

This pathway is shown in Fig. 17.1, whereby mild CKD progresses imperceptibly to kidney failure due to lack of measuring and monitoring kidney function in patients with recognized risks for CKD before they advance to symptomatic disease – the lack of a reliable early warning system. Too many CKD patients are first diagnosed after presenting with the clinical complications of kidney failure that require hospitalization with urgent hemodialysis catheter placement. This singular undesirable event frequently triggers a cascade of catheter-related bloodstream infections, repetitive hospital admissions, and antibiotic resistance. Such emergency management of patients with late-stage CKD is also costly, approximately $36,000 within the initial 3 months when urgent hemodialysis necessitates catheter placement rather than elective vascular access construction of an arteriovenous graft or fistula [9].

Implementing a Structured Approach to Improvement

The global strategy of our "Capturing Kidney Disease" program is depicted in Fig. 17.2. It mandated two philosophical principles of Japanese business: *kaizen* [10] and *monozukuri* [11]. *Kaizen* is the continuous quality improvement mantra of

OPTIMAL CKD SOLUTION

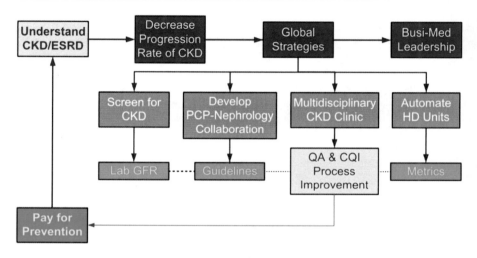

Fig. 17.2 Strategic plan to screen and optimize therapy of CKD in a multidisciplinary fashion that includes stakeholder involvement and process measurement and improvements. *ESRD* end-stage renal disease; *PCP* primary care physician; *HD* hemodialysis units; *GFR* glomerular filtration rate; *QA* quality assurance; *CQI* continuous quality improvement

Toyota Motor Corporation. *Monozukuri* means in simplistic terms, "the spirit to build excellent products and continually improve them." Instilling *kaizen* was the strategic step in our transformation, and the operational and tactical step was *monozukuri*. To realize our goal of rapidly accessible and system-wide CKD care, it would be necessary to construct an organized, web-enabled infrastructure of interacting computer databases to collect and deliver information to all nephrologists and, ultimately, to other collaborating providers through the electronic health record. Clinical decision support systems (CDSS) and computerized prescriber order entry (CPOE) systems would be particularly important to pursing *kaizen* and *monozukuri* (Table 17.1) [12].

The principles embedded in our strategy for developing and managing patient-centered CKD care were those also espoused by the "Six Sigma DMAIC" approach: define, measure, analyze, improve, and control [13, 14].

- Define: We would initially define the parameters of CKD and then target at-risk populations.
- Measure: Then, after such data acquisition, we would map our care and information flows, including communications to other healthcare providers. We would measure clinic interaction times, from the point of entry to the point of exit for typical patients, including time for providers to complete clinical documentation. Target outcomes of the National Kidney Foundation Kidney Disease Outcomes Quality Initiative (KDOQI™) Clinical Practice Guidelines (CPGs) [15] were also subjected to metric analysis at the provider level by provider type: staff physician,

Table 17.1 Components for reevaluation and reconstruction of clinical processes: definitions and requirements

Component	Meaning	Requirements
Kaizen	Philosophy of continuous quality improvement	Intense and concerted "buy in" and engagement
Monozukuri	Spirit to build things of high quality and to continually improve them	Key personnel and automation systems to develop infrastructure
DMAIC	Define, measure, analyze, improve, and control	Protocols to grade defined metrics, analysis tools, and dedicated team members to develop and implement consensus-based improvement and control processes
CDSS	Clinical decision support system	Evidence-based guidelines and review committees to determine components of implementation
CPOE	Computerized prescriber order entry (formerly "physician")	Distributed, robust, secure, automation infrastructure

fellow, and nurse practitioner. Patient satisfaction was measured independently by an external agency.

- Analyze and improve: Process efficiencies and bottlenecks were earmarked to streamline process flows and eliminate waste. Processes with the greatest variability were analyzed and corrected first. Practice homogeneity was our goal whenever possible, following the Pareto's principle: 80% of CKD patients would respond to highly protocolized care, and only 20% would require more individualistic therapeutic interventions [16]. One opportunity for standardization was laboratory ordering. Another was the evaluation of proteinuria.
- Control: Hopefully, these efforts would conclude with system developments that met their respective *takt* (cycle) times and led to zero work in progress (WIP) [17].

We defined WIP from the time a patient was seen until the time that all nephrology and multidisciplinary care relevant to CKD was completed, including the point at which all communications and health record entries had been received and acted upon. This WIP time was substantially greater than the point-of-care time alone. This definition continuously drove providers to complete their clinical cycle times as rapidly as possible and to create a continuous communications environment with PCPs and patients. In addition, more rapid clinical documentation would improve the revenue cycle.

While producing a decrease in WIP, we established a concurrent goal of improving patient access to the CKD clinic. To achieve these potentially competing goals, clinic visit times were reduced by one-third: 60-min new patient referrals and consultations would be conducted within 40 and 30-min follow-up visits were shortened to 20 min. Our assumption was that CKD is complex for patients, and therefore, that presenting information for longer periods would not be fruitful. We would instead strive to have the patients' problem(s) and education more sharply focused.

Table 17.2 The five stages of chronic kidney disease (CKD)

Stage 1	eGFR greater than 90 mL/min with some sign of kidney damage on other tests
Stage 2	eGFR of 60–90 mL/min with some signs of kidney damage (if eGFR is 60 mL/min or greater with no other signs of kidney damage, there is no CKD)
Stage 3	eGFR of 30–59 mL/min, a moderate reduction in kidney function
Stage 4	eGFR of 15–29 mL/min, a severe reduction in kidney function
Stage 5	eGFR less than 15 mL/min, established kidney failure, renal replacement treatment may be needed

Such concise and precise communication was required to establish and realize the NKF KDOQI™ CPGs [15]. It was deemed better to be direct and brief and to have the patient return for a second round of care and education, than to try to "cram everything into" a single office visit.

Action Plans and Operational Changes

Ensuring our providers' knowledge base. Enacting this strategy would require multiple tactics and operational changes. We first had to renew and standardize our expertise in CKD. This effort focused on our becoming highly familiar with the NKF KDOQI™ CPGs that had been released several months before our project was launched. These guidelines were predicated on the best available evidence upon which all of us could center our practices, globally strategize our care, and hopefully mitigate CKD progression in the Henry Ford patient population.

An early warning system for CKD – focusing on the eGFR. We first would need to develop an early warning system of CKD. For this, we worked with the clinical laboratory of our healthcare system to implement the Modification of Diet in Renal Disease eGFR as a standard measure of kidney function and the backbone of our efforts [18]. We further defined the "*e*" of eGFR as not only estimated, but also "electronic."

The eGFR, for those readers less familiar with how the kidney functions, is a measure of how well an individual's kidneys are filtering wastes from the blood into the urine, expressed as the milliliters of blood filtered per minute. The lower the kidney's function, the lower the eGFR. It is calculated from a blood test for creatinine – a waste product of muscle cells, and a patient's age, gender, and race. The eGFR value defines normal kidney function and the various stages of CKD, as Table 17.2 summarizes.

Our intent was to publish the eGFR with each outpatient serum creatinine ordered by Henry Ford providers as a first step. Prior to activating this system-wide eGFR reporting initiative, our nephrologists worked closely with internists and family practitioners in a variety of educational formats to assure their effective interpretation of this new and more informative laboratory report. Before we began routine reporting of the *e*GFR with the serum creatinine in 2002, nearly 3 of 4 CKD consultations were for patients with *e*GFRs lower than 45 mL/min/1.73 m². In such patients, cardiovascular events rise steeply [19].

Over the following 3 years, the distribution of *e*GFRs at first presentation to the CKD Clinic shifted to earlier stages, such that only 11% of referrals were at stage 5, a testament to widespread *e*GFR publication and provider education. Intervening earlier in the course of patients' CKD not only reduced the rate of disease progression in many, but also provided positive impacts on the management of patients whose CKD did continue to progress.

Increasing access to care. To address the increased size of our CKD clinic population, we formulated strategies to increase patient access, pilot tested them, and implemented improvements. One of these was a "just say yes" scheduling policy that decreased average outpatient clinic access to just 48 h for new consultations. Direct communication between the referring physician and a nephrologist was the only requirement prior to scheduling the clinic visit.

Strengthening provider and patient education. Attenuating CKD progression provided a more extended opportunity for patient education; however, this was no longer provided by physicians, but in a structured format by those who interacted most frequently with patients: nurses, dialysis technicians, dietitians, pharmacists, and social workers. As one result, physicians experienced a "gain in time" that contributed to our previously mentioned increased patient visit capacity. As another, the proportion of our late-stage CKD population who choose transplantation and peritoneal dialysis, rather than hemodialysis for renal replacement therapy, increased from 10 to 38% over 7 years, and temporary hemodialysis catheter insertions were supplanted by safer, higher quality tunneled, cuffed-catheter procedures.

Although *e*GFR dissemination was successful, it produced an increase in low value nephrology consultations for patients with *e*GFRs in the high CKD stage 3 range, 45–59 mL/min. Targeted PCP and patient education gradually addressed this "worried well" referral problem by providing reassurance and encouraging PCPs to provide regular monitoring and risk factor management instead of requesting consultation.

We also repackaged the NKF CPGs into a small booklet of digestible CKD morsels of knowledge [20]. All the participant stakeholders requested such guidance [21]. The booklet has aligned and harmonized our CKD program with our referring PCPs for the first time. The seven modules (Fig. 17.3) include cardiovascular risk factor modification through controlling blood sugar, lipids, and hypertension; proteinuria reduction; evaluation of CKD progression; vaccinations/immunizations; nutritional assessment; anemia management; and CKD-mineral and bone disorder management (CKD-MBD) [22]. The latter includes submodules on vitamin D deficiency, metabolic acidosis, renal osteodystrophy, and secondary hyperparathyroidism. The booklet also contains a checklist of CKD "things to do," based on our belief that a checklist would increase the likelihood of the multiple care goals of a CKD patient being met.

However, patients also required other, more specific educational resources to achieve success. For those with lesser degrees of CKD, we provided professionally written "take home" materials, designed for our socioeconomically disadvantaged

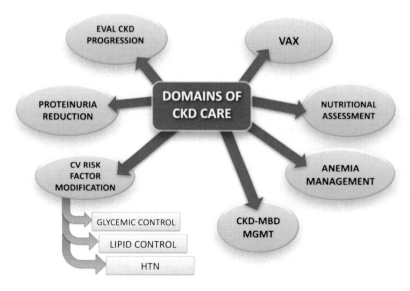

Fig. 17.3 CKD represented as a 7-disease domain complex

patient population. We then ensured that the materials actually left the office for "at home reading." We also enlisted patient education experts to develop a CKD Education Class for patients with Stage 3B CKD, or worse. Such classes had been shown to reduce urgent dialysis therapy [23]. A free weekly class was also designed for patients with nonresolving acute kidney injury and their families to teach the nutritional and social aspects of CKD, the various types of renal replacement therapy, and how this information would be useful for those whose disease would progress. With time, this patient-centered education had a profound effect: the proportion of patients electing peritoneal dialysis steadily increased to 38%, a nearly unbelievable circumstance.

For quick reference, the CKD booklet also contained evidence-based algorithms for each CKD domain of care. Ultimately, this "playbook" was distributed on the healthcare system's intranet and was made instantly accessible as a "menu" item within the healthcare record. A printed version that fit comfortably in the clinician's white coat pocket was delivered to healthcare providers. Multiple other healthcare groups have requested this popular publication, and it has provided the template for the Michigan Quality Initiative Consortium's annual CKD guidelines and the National Kidney Foundation of Illinois' CPGs.

Redesigning Our CKD Clinic

1. Facilities and Personnel: Our now reconstructed CKD clinic has six examination rooms; dedicated patient-level appropriate literature regarding CKD-specific drugs, diabetes, kidney stones, and hypertension; one dedicated procedure room

for intravenous fluid and iron infusions; and a clinical laboratory. It houses an invigorated nurse manager and her staff, a pharmacist, a social worker, a renal nutritionist, two adult nurse practitioners, and a clinical laboratory technician. All tests necessary for optimal patient management are provided within 20 min – urinalysis, urine protein-to-creatinine ratio, serum electrolytes, blood urea nitrogen, serum creatinine, glucose, calcium, phosphorus, and albumin. The nurse practitioners and pharmacist were the only new additions to the clinic, but the workflows of the physicians, other healthcare providers, and staff were optimized to expedite patients' care. This multidisciplinary, standardized approach guided by the NKF KDOQI™ CPGs reduced clinic visit time and produced an 8% improvement in patient satisfaction within just 6 months, as measured by a recognized, national survey.

2. Management: One staff physician is held accountable for administering the CKD Clinic each day. His/her duties include supervising the nurse practitioners and nephrology fellows, providing "urgent" consultations, resolving differences between patients and providers or other personnel, and being accountable for any and all procedures and laboratory tests conducted during the clinic. The managing physician's assuring other physicians' adherence to appointment times reduced waiting-room time, and not surprisingly, patient complaints regarding "wait times."

3. Financial planning: We realized early on that redesign of our clinic would require money and financial planning. We anticipated that hiring an additional nurse practitioner and a pharmacist would improve clinic access, reduce medication-related errors, and provide other care synergies, but that investing in these resources would require "lean" budgeting. We recognized that improving our inventory management and reducing expenses were important, but that increased billing would be the ultimate driver of success and staying within our budget.

4. Standardizing billing and coding: Although there are many parts of the revenue cycle, the most important for clinicians are optimal coding and preventing rejections/denials. We documented our billing inefficiencies and challenged our group to succeed in this area. Education by our divisional and healthcare system's billing managers increased our knowledge of the processes involved. We sampled the clinical encounters of approximately 100 patients to determine which diagnoses appeared most frequently. These were graphed, and an "optical mark reader" billing sheet was constructed. Diagnoses were matched to exact ICD-9-CM codes and were mapped to a billable code.

5. Standardizing clinical documentation: Employing clear, concise, and precise language in clinical documentation was also paramount. "Hypertension" was now always "benign" or "malignant" high blood pressure. CKD stages were consistently coded. Primary diagnoses were coded first. In addition, when conducting the nephrology fellows' mentored CKD clinic, we often reversed the traditional paradigm of clinical presentation followed by billing. The "billing sheet" was presented first, and the fellow's presentation was required to justify the billing. Moreover, each patient's CKD education was standardized and documented. We taught clinical nephrology such that the NKF CPGs would be promoted and applied to patient care, with areas of controversy discussed in a

scholarly manner. Concomitantly, data collection was refocused on measuring clinical targets in the processes and outcomes of care, permitting objective feedback to trainees. Our emphasis on the NKF KDOQI CPGs improved teaching of core knowledge in this burgeoning area of medicine.

Initially, and as expected, mismatches occurred between billing and documentation. With time, however, the fellows more clearly understood these discrepancies, and the billing cycle improved by identifying errors promptly and reconciling them before charge submission, thereby reducing our most controllable and worst revenue cycle bottleneck. Billing throughput increased, as did cash flows. Biller "stress" was alleviated, and their work was shifted to improving other areas of the billing cycle. These improvement projects enhanced the quality of the fellows' clinical documentation and fulfilled the Accreditation Council for Graduate Medical Education's requirement that supervisory staff prepare fellows for the business and practice of nephrology.

In summary, coupled with increased visit capacity, our improved billing efficiency increased revenues by 35% over 2 years through a disciplined, collective effort. Two new positions were supported, better patient access was achieved, clinic patient cycle times were reduced, and clinical documentation was improved.

6. Improving Communications with Our Referring Physicians. We also developed a multidisciplinary approach to changing the communication flow with PCPs following patient encounters [24–27]. This would ultimately decrease the number of informational transactions for patients and between providers, improve the completing of necessary work, and reduce miscommunication(s). For example, a nephrologist evaluating a patient with proteinuria for whom no anti-renin-angiotensin-aldosterone-system antagonist had been prescribed would now prescribe one of these agents, rather than suggesting that the referring physician do so. The electronic or paper communication back to the PCP would indicate that the appropriate agent had been initiated, that it should be escalated within certain constraints by the PCP, and that the nephrologist was at-the-ready for any questions regarding subsequent kidney-relevant care. Sustaining this process would establish and document an essential, evidence-based treatment for the patient and avoid a call to the PCP to start the drug. The prescriptions were generated electronically through a statewide pharmacy system in most cases, facilitating medication reconciliation among all involved parties.

We expanded our CKD program's educational initiatives to PCP's by preparing illustrative clinical cases and sending them to PCP group leaders by email. Each case demonstrated in a nonpejorative tone how one or two pieces of evidence-based nephrology could be utilized. Links to source material, including our own CKD booklet, were provided. These miniature "educational moments" were well received, and they were supplemented by annual symposia that updated the current state of knowledge in CKD through analyzing a complex CKD case. A patient with hypertension, anemia, depressed serum bicarbonate concentration, vascular calcification, and secondary hyperparathyroidism would be presented, and managing hypertension, the progression of CKD, anemia of CKD management, and CKD-MBD (CKD-Mineral and Bone Disorder) would be discussed.

7. Addressing Patients' Comorbidities. CKD patients at higher risk for influenza and pneumococcal pneumonia received their annual influenza vaccinations at the CKD Clinic, if these had not already been administered, beginning in early autumn, and these services were documented in the electronic health record. Patients were saved a separate visit to the PCP and efficiency was increased across our healthcare continuum [26, 28]. This approach produced a marked improvement, even though only 57% accepted immunization, from our 0% historical control. Most importantly, the proportion of CKD stage 4 and 5 patients at risk for hepatitis B virus who were immunized before the initiation of renal replacement therapy increased substantially. This is critical because patients' response to immunization declines significantly with advancing kidney failure [29].

This multidisciplinary, proactive approach has been successful in our program and elsewhere. A comparative trial between Eastern and Western Canada pitted traditional vs. multidisciplinary care in CKD patients with progressive disease. The Western Canadian approach of multidisciplinary care proved superior for survivorship after the initiation of hemodialysis, suggesting that a healthier patient entering the hemodialysis center would fare better than a less healthy one.

8. Building an Electronic Clinical Database, CDSS, and CPOE. To efficiently carry out our mission, we required a new electronic informational infrastructure. Otherwise, information outflow would consume more provider and staff resources and decrease productivity. An enhanced computer database would also be required to measure performance and guide our group's continuous practice and outcomes improvement initiatives. We reasoned that if these new tactics could be carefully implemented, any future "pay for performance" metrics would have already been established or could be easily added.

Our first database was a standardized clinic visit note embedded within a front-end interface that became the cornerstone of our nurse practitioners' practices. This web-enabled clinical tool employed various reminders in each CKD domain of care (Fig. 17.2). It was synchronized with the CKD booklet checklists and algorithms. It prompted timely and cogent documentation and coalesced all of the manual input into an attractive note-report that was uploaded into the health record. Synergy between the nurse practitioners who utilized this CKD-specific database and billers contributed to reduced payment rejections. PCP groups appreciated these concise, precise, direct, and predictable reports.

Furthermore, patient weight, blood pressure, and other parameters could be "pulled" from the healthcare system database and analyzed. For example, review of blood pressure control by our CKD nurse practitioners revealed that 75% of patients had achieved a systolic blood pressure of 140 mmHg or less, and 52% 130 mmHg or less – better than national data for blood pressure control in hypertensive individuals among the general population. Control of intact parathyroid hormone testing to NKF CPG levels was also exemplary. Concomitant improvements in vaccination rates and vitamin D levels were also achieved, and there was a 25% improvement in the use of anti-renin-angiotensin-aldosterone medications.

Harkening back to the CKD booklet's checklist, the CKD clinic database also facilitated trend analysis of care by individual providers [23]. Clinical treatments could be correlated with outcomes. All parameters that were not at their respective target were addressed. Repetitive trend analyses produced an expected regression to the mean, and individual patients and populations of all providers achieved a positive impact on global CKD care.

A CPOE with CDSS was then conceived and implemented for patients with the anemia of CKD. Before deployment of this computerized anemia management program (CAMP©) [30], all physicians were paged regarding erythropoiesis-stimulating agent (ESA) dosing of their anemic patients, frequently disrupting clinical work and leading to hasty dosing without the benefit of trend analysis. This anemia-based CPOE was algorithm and query-based, and web-enabled. It was formulated to incorporate best practices for anemia management informed by large clinical trials [31–33], and with the following goals: reducing the time to administer ESAs; extending the dosing interval between ESA injections to once monthly; providing timely clinical documentation; providing ESA dosing and ferrokinetic trend analysis; and improving patient safety by warning the provider of supratherapeutic ESA dosing. European nephrology-anemia experts had also considered such a system [34]. This algorithm would also provide monthly ESA treatment with darbepoetin to any patient who required ESA therapy, regardless of prior ESA exposure.

Standardized documentation mandated input of patient demographics, iron parameters, hemoglobin; provider; ESA type and dose; iron type (oral or intravenous) and dose; site of injection; and, importantly, a checkbox that indicated that the patient had received counseling regarding drug(s) administration. All of these data fed a back-end database, providing the substrate for individual- and group-level statistical analysis. Moreover, the form was forwarded for review and electronic signature to the patient's original ESA-ordering nephrologist.

By having real-time right-of-passage to the entirety of the data regarding ESA administration, inventory management and control of intravenous iron and ESA improved, as did cash flows. Patient throughput within the clinic increased as the *takt* time for ESA administration plummeted nearly 85%. When an injection was given, the clinical documentation followed promptly. The net results of management by CAMP© were mean reductions in ESA dosing at the patient and group levels; homogeneously increased iron utilization by either oral or intravenous routes, with the pharmaco-economic benefit of overall reduction in ESA utilization; and real-time documentation that augmented and synergized our billing procedures [35].

The CAMP© software, effectively and without provider intervention, attained NKF KDOQI™ CPG-based anemia targets in 80% of anemic CKD individuals by 5–6 months, while reducing ESA agent reimbursement times. It permitted a deep "drill-down" of the roughly 10% of individuals who had experienced a suboptimal result with CAMP© or were requiring higher dosing and were therefore considered ESA hypo-responders from whichever cause. Individuals were identified with absolute and/or functional iron deficiency, undiagnosed inflammatory conditions that induced bone marrow hypo-responsiveness, covert bleeding, and providers who had overridden internal system logic. Again, Pareto's principle was confirmed by our ability to separate routine and exceptional patients. Lastly, congruent with the notion that patient safety is at the core of any

CDSS, CAMP© alerted physicians in text and graphics on desktop computers or mobile platforms of any untoward trends in their patients' anemia management, including iron deficiency and rapid hemoglobin declines or elevations. These warnings could easily be retransmitted to PCPs by email or via the electronic health record.

Building upon the successes of our automation processes, we extended CDSS and CPOE into other realms of CKD care. We deployed an inpatient consultation database that notified physicians of "the what, when, why, and where" of their hospitalized patients. We also developed systems to monitor vascular accesses in patients undergoing hemodialysis. This provided an independently validated early warning system to prevent vascular access occlusion by thrombosis [36], a clinical and economic nightmare comparable to hemodialysis catheter-related blood stream infections. Lastly, we have begun to rationalize the multiple processes involved in providing inpatient renal replacement therapies in various formats. If successful, all providers will be able to electronically track CKD patients throughout our healthcare system.

Conclusion

A change in our *mien* has truly changed the mean of our clinical practice from high variability, and to some extent, unreliable clinical and business outcomes. This metamorphosis has required self-evaluation and reflection, then adhering to a "lean" clinical operational approach that defines, measures, analyzes, improves, and controls clinical processes in order to augment their results. Over the course of our journey, we have accomplished increased patient access and improved patient satisfaction; increased clinical revenues that have supported new assets and personnel to provide more comprehensive and a higher level of care; improved clinical documentation; increased billing efficiency; improved collaboration with our PCP colleagues; and algorithm-directed, patient-centered, multidisciplinary care. We have achieved these improvements through strategic planning and assiduous labor, while adhering to the precepts of *kaizen*, *monozukuri*, and acknowledging Pareto's principle.

We have implemented CDSS and CPOE with modular, extensible databases from which clinical outcomes can be gleaned, analyzed, and improved. Remarkably, as a follow-on, the group generated sufficient momentum to reach into the community of Detroit; we initiated nurse practitioner outreach to screen for CKD, including diabetes, hypertension, and proteinuria patients who do not realize the extent of their as-yet asymptomatic problems. In addition, we participated in nearly every major State of Michigan- or National Kidney Foundation of Michigan CKD-related event. These events included several federally funded programs targeting obesity, hypertension, and the continuum of CKD, from screening asymptomatic persons and their relatives to kidney allograft recipients. By breaking out of our "ivory tower," we have been able to extend our brand name and assist in the generating of a future healthier community. Throughout our reincarnation, our outcomes and achievements have been reported and recognized, first locally, then regionally and, finally, nationally.

Although our journey is far from over, it becomes difficult to remember 8 years later where we once were. Yet our visitors remind us frequently of the aspects of our CKD Clinic that differentiate us from others. Thus, we conclude with a *haiku* by the samurai poet Masahide, a disciple of Basho, who in 1688 declared: "Barn's burnt down – now, I can see the moon" [37, 38].

Editor's Comments: I asked a nephrologist colleague, Dr. Bryan Becker, who he would suggest as the best CKD management example for our book. He responded, "Jerry Yee." No wonder! The Henry Ford nephrology team's story is continuous improvement methodology at its best, and their results show it. Deming took this approach to Japan in the 50's. Henry Ford nephrology has applied Toyota's methods – terminology and all, and with stunning successes within a difficult-to-manage urban patient population. Their emphasis on preparing trainees for effective practice within the outpatient practice environment is notable. JTH

Acknowledgments: The authors extend their gratitude for the expert reading and critique of the manuscript by Ms. Livia Berardi and Mr. James Kelly.

References

1. http://quickfacts.census.gov/qfd/states/26/2622000.html. Accessed 6 Dec 2010.
2. http://www.worldhealth.net/news/detroit_takes_title_of_fattest_city_from/. Accessed 6 Dec 2010.
3. U.S. Renal Data System: USRDS 2004 annual data report. Bethesda: National Institutes of Health, National Institute of Diabetes and Digestive and Kidney Diseases www.usrds.org/adr_2004.htm.
4. McCullough PA, Vassalotti JA, Collins AJ, Chen SC, Bakris GL. National Kidney Foundation's Kidney Early Evaluation Program (KEEP) annual data report 2009: executive summary. Am J Kidney Dis. 2010;55(3 Suppl 2):S1–3.
5. Levey AS, Bosch JP, Lewis JB, Greene T, Rogers N, Roth D. A more accurate method to estimate glomerular filtration rate from serum creatinine: a new prediction equation. Modification of Diet in Renal Disease Study Group. Ann Intern Med. 1999;130:461–70.
6. Coresh J, Selvin E, Stevens LA, Manzi J, Kusek JW, Eggers P, et al. Prevalence of chronic kidney disease in the United States. JAMA. 2007;298(17):2038–47.
7. Levin A, Chaudhry MR, Djurdjev O, Beaulieu M, Komenda P. Diabetes, kidney disease and cardiovascular disease patients. Assessing care of complex patients using outpatient testing and visits: additional metrics by which to evaluate health care system functioning. Nephrol Dial Transplant. 2009;24:2714–20.
8. Thanamayooran S, Rose C, Hirsch DJ. Effectiveness of a multidisciplinary kidney disease clinic in achieving treatment guideline targets. Nephrol Dial Transplant. 2005;20:2385–93.
9. St. Peter WL, et al. Chronic kidney disease: the distribution of health care dollars. Kidney Int. 2004;66:313–21.
10. Jacobson GH, McCoin NS, Lescallette R, Russ S, Slovis CM. Kaizen: a method of process improvement in the emergency department. Acad Emerg Med. 2009;16(12):1341–9.
11. Oshima S. History of homegrown Japanese science finally adds up. Japan Times. Sunday, 10 Aug 2003.

12. Finlay DD, Nugent CD, Wang H, Donnelly MP, McCullagh PJ. Mining, knowledge and decision support. Technol Health Care. 2010;18(6):429–41.
13. Brue G, Howes R. The McGraw-Hill 36-hour course: six sigma. Chapter 1: introduction to six sigma. New York: McGraw-Hill; 2006. p. 9.
14. http://www.sixsigmaspc.com/dictionary/DMAIC-definemeasureanalyzeimprovecontrol.html. Accessed 30 Nov 2010.
15. http://www.kidney.org/professionals/KDOQI/guidelines_ckd/toc.htm. Accessed 25 Sept 2011.
16. Brue G, Howes R. The McGraw-Hill 36-hour course: six sigma. Chapter 7: define phase. New York: McGraw-Hill; 2006. p. 148.
17. http://en.wikipedia.org/wiki/Takt_time. Accessed 4 Dec 2010.
18. Levey AS, Coresh J, Greene T, Marsh J, Stevens LA, Kusek JW, Van Lente F; Chronic Kidney Disease Epidemiology Collaboration. Expressing the modification of diet in renal disease study equation for estimating glomerular filtration rate with standardized serum creatinine values. Clin Chem. 2007;53(4):766–72.
19. Go AS, et al. Chronic kidney disease and risks of death, cardiovascular events, and hospitalization. New Engl J Med. 2004;351:1296–1305.
20. http://www.ghsrenal.com. Accessed 3 Dec 2010.
21. Boulware LE, et al. Identification and referral of patients with progressive CKD: a national study. Am J Kidney Dis. 2006;48(2):192–204.
22. Kidney Disease: Improving Global Outcomes (KDIGO) CKD-MBD Work Group. KDIGO clinical practice guideline for the diagnosis, evaluation, prevention, and treatment of chronic kidney disease-mineral and bone disorder (CKD-MBD). Kidney Int Suppl. 2009;113:S1–30.
23. Van Biesen W, Verbeke F, Vanholder R. We don't need no education… (Pink Floyd, The Wall). Multidisciplinary predialysis education programmes: pass or fail? Nephrol Dial Transplant. 2009;24:3277–9.
24. Goldstein M, et al. Multidisciplinary predialysis care and morbidity of patients on dialysis. Am J Kidney Dis. 2004;44:70614.
25. Hemmelgarn BR, Manns BJ, Zhang J, Tonelli M, Klarenbach S, Walsh M, Culleton BF, for the Alberta Kidney Disease Network. Association between multidisciplinary care and survival for elderly patients with chronic kidney disease. J Am Soc Nephrol. 2007;18:993–9.
26. Dinits-Pensy M, et al. The use of vaccine in adult patients with renal disease. Adv Chronic Kidney Dis. 2005;46:997–1011.
27. Curtis BM, Ravani P, Malberti F, et al. The short- and long-term impact of multi-disciplinary clinics in addition to standard nephrology care on patient outcomes. Nephrol Dial Transplant. 2005;20:147–54.
28. http://www.cdc.gov/mmwr/preview/mmwrhtml/rr5416a1.htm. Accessed 29 Nov 2010.
29. Litjens NH, et al. Impaired immune responses and antigen-specific CD4+ T cells in hemodialysis patients. J Am Soc Nephrol. 2088;19:1483–90.
30. Chalhoub E, Ismail K, Yee J, Frinak S. CAMP: a continuous quality initiative control tool. J Clin Nephrol., accepted for publication.
31. Pfeffer M, Burdmann EA, Cooper DE, et al. A trial of darbepoetin alfa in type 2 diabetes and chronic kidney disease. N Engl J Med. 2009;361:1–14.
32. Singh AK, Szczech L, Tang KL, et al. CHOIR Investigators. Correction of anemia with epoetin alfa in chronic kidney disease. N Engl J Med. 2006;355:2085–98.
33. Drüeke TB, Locatelli F, Clyne N, et al. CREATE Investigators. Normalization of hemoglobin level in patients with chronic kidney disease and anemia. N Engl J Med. 2006;355:2071–84.
34. Goldsmith D, Covic A. Time to Reconsider Evidence for Anaemia Treatment (TREAT)= Essential Safety Arguments (ESA). Nephrol Dial Transplant. 2010;25:1734–7.
35. Besarab A, Frinak S, Yee J. An indistinct balance: the safety and efficacy of parenteral iron therapy. J Am Soc Nephrol. 1999;10:2029–43.
36. Frinak S, Zasuwa G, Dunfee T, Besarab A, Yee J. Dynamic venous access pressure ratio test for hemodialysis access monitoring. Am J Kidney Dis. 2002;40(4) 760–8.
37. Gallagher J. Reimagining Detroit, Time Magazine, vol. 176. http://www.time.com/time/nation/article/0,8599,2030766,00.html. Accessed 11 Nov 2010.
38. http://www.ict.ne.jp/~basho-bp. Accessed 4 Dec 2010.

Chapter 18
Asthma: Identifying and Treating High-Risk Patients

Michael B. Foggs

Keywords Asthma • Guidelines • Stepwise • High-risk • Anticipatory Asthma Care • Advocate Health Care • Urban

Asthma is a generic, wastebasket term. It includes a group of complex, chronic inflammatory, multidimensional, markedly heterogeneous lung diseases that are similar enough to be lumped under the rubric "asthma." This chapter summarizes our incomplete understandings about the causes, the disordered physiology, and the clinical variability of asthma; the principles of its diagnosis and treatment; and the need to move from usual to anticipatory care for best short- and long-term patient outcomes and costs. I will spend considerable space discussing asthma risk, severity, control, and treatment responsiveness because these concepts interact in guiding asthma management for individual patients and populations. I conclude by describing a system-based approach we have developed at Advocate Health Care that has improved outcomes for our urban patients with high-risk asthma (Fig. 18.1).

What Do We Know About Asthma?

The causes of asthma are poorly understood, and are undoubtedly multidimensional. Asthma exacerbations, commonly known as "attacks" or "flares", are one of its hallmarks, and constitute its major ominous outcome, short of mortality. Asthma exacerbations reflect intense inflammation of the lungs induced by one or more triggers. While each trigger may act through a different mechanism, the endpoint is multicellular

M.B. Foggs, MD (✉)
Allergy/Immunology, Advocate Health Care, Chicago, IL, USA
e-mail: immunotype@aol.com

J.T. Harrington and E.D. Newman (eds.), *Great Health Care: Making It Happen*,
DOI 10.1007/978-1-4614-1198-7_18, © Springer Science+Business Media, LLC 2012

Fig. 18.1 Michael B. Foggs, MD

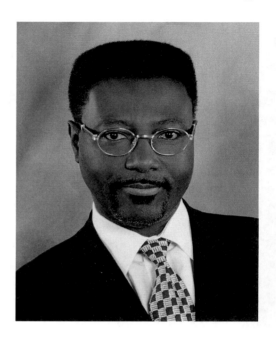

inflammation, enhanced bronchial hyperresponsiveness, and airflow obstruction. The symptoms are cough and breathing difficulty. This event can be fatal. By definition there is no such thing as a mild asthma exacerbation [1]. It is critical for healthcare providers to accurately assess the severity of asthma exacerbations [2], and for patients to understand their significance (Fig. 18.2) [1].

Asthma expression among patients is variable due to gene-environment interactions, multiple pathophysiological mechanisms, varied environmental exposures, comorbidities, age, underlying disease severity, inconsistencies in healthcare access, the quality of care received, psychosocial factors, responsiveness to asthma therapy, and the burden of comorbid diseases. Simple as all that! Recent gene cluster analysis shows that this syndrome has multiple phenotypes (variations in its clinical expression) [3]. The demographics of asthma patients combined with these expressed phenotypes primarily define subgroups at high risk for poor asthma outcomes, and the many other risk factors just mentioned also contribute to the patient's likelihood of exacerbations, premature loss of lung function, and death.

These high-risk asthmatics need to be identified, especially African–Americans and Puerto Ricans, since their bronchial inflammation is disproportionately high in comparison to others. In keeping with individualized therapy, aggressive interventions should relate not only to the patient's current impairment, but also to their ethnicity, in order to minimize unfavorable outcomes and reduce medical resource utilization.

	Symptoms and Signs	Initial PEF (or FEV1)	Clinical Course
Mild	Dyspnea only with activity (assess tachypnea in young children)	PEF ≥ 70 percent predicted or personal best	■ Usually cared for at home ■ Prompt relief with inhaled SABA ■ Possible short course of oral systemic corticosteroids
Moderate	Dyspnea interferes with or limits usual activity	PEF 40–69 percent predicted or personal best	■ Usually requires office or ED visit ■ Relief from frequent inhaled SABA ■ Oral systemic corticosteroids; some symptoms last for 1–2 days after treatment is begun
Severe	Dyspnea at rest; interferes with conversation	PEF <40 percent predicted or personal best	■ Usually requires ED visit and likely hospitalization ■ Partial relief from frequent inhaled SABA ■ Oral systemic corticosteroids; some symptoms last for >3 days after treatment is begun ■ Adjunctive therapies are helpful
Subset: Life threatening	Too dyspneic to speak; perspiring	PEF <25 percent predicted or personal best	■ Requires ED/hospitalization; possible ICU ■ Minimal or no relief from frequent inhaled SABA ■ Intravenous corticosteroids ■ Adjunctive therapies are helpful

Key: ED, emergency department; FEV_1, forced expiratory volume in 1 second; ICU, intensive care unit; PEF, peak expiratory flow; SABA, short-acting beta$_2$-agonist

Fig. 18.2 Classifying the severity of asthma exacerbations in an emergency setting

Diagnosing and Managing Asthma

Underdiagnosis and late diagnosis are common, especially in inner-city populations, which have an excess of high-risk individuals to begin with [4]. How can asthma so often advance to become a high-risk disease before it is diagnosed? In fact, symptoms are frequently ignored or blamed on a common cold or poor physical conditioning, especially when the patient is obese as well. The waxing and waning symptoms of asthma are not recognized as due to persisting lung inflammation. The diagnosis must be suspected clinically because there is no diagnostic blood test for asthma. Under these circumstances, lung inflammation smolders and escalates, even causing permanent damage before anti-inflammatory therapy is finally started.

Within the Advocate Health Care system we adhere strongly to the National Heart, Lung, and Blood Institute (NHLBI)/National Asthma Education Prevention Program (NAEPP) "Guidelines for the Diagnosis and Management of Asthma [1]." The asthma clinical practice guidelines provide a necessary framework for this individualized therapy, because retrospective analysis has demonstrated that their use:

1. Improves quality of care and outcomes
2. Decreases unnecessary and inappropriate practice variations
3. Decreases healthcare costs
4. Fosters evidence-based decision-making
5. Accelerates the application and translation of advances in medical science to everyday clinical practice, especially in large medical practices [5].

At the same time, we are cautious to individualize therapy based on direct assessment, clinician judgment, and patient preferences.

Managing asthma requires assessment along several parameters – severity, control, impairment, and risk. While earlier guidelines stressed the importance of classifying "asthma severity", the current NHLBI guidelines provide a renewed focus on "asthma control." This new paradigm characterizes both severity and control within the context of past and current impairment of lung function, and current and future risks for exacerbations and further impairment. It can be effectively applied to both high-risk inner-city asthma patients and the wide spectrum of patients in other varied healthcare delivery environments. It is also important to understand that interventions may not improve both current impairment and future risk in parallel, particularly for high-risk inner-city patients who are impacted by many unpredictable variables that continue to place them at high risk, no matter how well they are doing at any point in time.

From this perspective, evaluating current impairment includes:

- Assessing daytime and nighttime symptoms
- Assessing the need for quick-relief short acting β-agonists
- Objectively measuring lung function, (i.e., spirometry)
- Assessing tolerated activity level
- Assessing quality of life
- Assessing the patient's satisfaction with the partnership and asthma care provided by their clinician

The asthma guidelines strongly recommend the use of validated questionnaires to assess impairment whenever possible in both children and adults with asthma.

Assessing future asthma risk is a different matter. This encompasses a broader evaluation of the patient's past medical history and current asthma disposition, (e.g., history of exacerbations, risk of premature loss of lung function or reduced lung growth in children, ethnicity, and risk of medication side-effects). Both the frequency and severity of past exacerbations are important. For example, a person who has experienced one severe exacerbation within the past year may have a greater risk of experiencing a future life-threatening attack than a person who has experienced two or more moderate exacerbations during the same period of time.

The asthma guidelines recommend further that physicians consider both the patient's short-term (past 4 weeks) and long-term or global (past 12 months) histories in assessing both "asthma severity" and "asthma control." Asthma severity should be assessed before starting treatment, whether in a newly diagnosed patient or in an established patient being evaluated by a clinician for the first time. It should then be revisited only rarely because it often changes with time – spontaneously, as a result of exposure to or avoidance of asthma triggers, or as a result of implementing or withdrawing therapy. As a result, its use is limited for choosing treatments and predicting response [6, 7]. For example, it is obvious that a person who requires only one anti-inflammatory medication to establish optimal control has less severe asthma than a chronic persistent asthmatic who achieves equal control, but requires three or more long-term medications to do so.

In contrast, "asthma control" provides a more meaningful assessment of impairment and risk over time. Continually assessing each patient's asthma based on control instead of severity, and using the paradigm of *current impairment* and *future risk*, provides the best guidance for therapy. This is a complex challenge for the patient and the clinical team, since there is no single means to achieving asthma control. A variety of contributors are important: confirming the diagnosis, providing the correct asthma treatment, the patient's adhering to treatment and proper use of inhaler devices, avoiding allergens and irritants, and diagnosis and treatment of any comorbidities that may aggravate, or masquerade as asthma. And in the end, well-controlled asthma does not necessarily imply mild asthma, and poorly controlled asthma does not necessarily imply severe asthma.

Stepwise Asthma Care

Responsiveness to therapy is the ease with which a patient's asthma is controlled. Responsiveness varies, even among patients with asthma of similar severity. Responsiveness appears to be impacted strongly by pharmacogenetics and pharmacogenomics – each patient's unique underlying genetic and chemical makeup, but exactly how these impact any individual's response to a variety of asthma treatments is only partially understood at this time.

Individualized management requires a stepwise approach to gain and maintain control in both the impairment and risk domains. The primary objective is to bring asthma under control in an efficient and safe manner. An additional goal is to maintain asthma control with the least number and amount of medications, and thereby, minimize the risk of adverse effects. The level of control achieved will ultimately guide decisions about adjusting therapy over time.

Unfortunately, we have no truly curative asthma medicines. Inflammation and airways hyperresponsiveness recur upon withdrawal of long-term anti-inflammatory therapy in patients with chronic persistent asthma [8]. Asthma is also poorly controlled in some patients even if they adhere to their prescribed treatments, and successfully avoid environmental asthma triggers. A better understanding of asthma's causes will be required to address these shortcomings of current treatments, but these shortcomings do not imply that treatments are not improving or that they do not reduce impairment and improve risk for most patients.

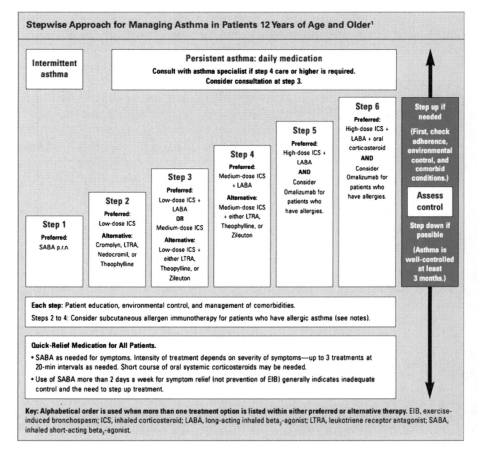

Fig. 18.3 Stepwise approach for managing asthma in youths ≥12 years of age and adults

The "stepwise approach" operates on the premise that the dose, number of medications, and frequency of administration should be increased as the situation dictates and decreased whenever this can be accomplished safely: step up if necessary, step down if possible (Fig. 18.3) [1]. Therapy for chronic persistent asthma must attempt to not only improve current control, but also reduce inflammatory foci throughout the airways over the long-term, preventing or decreasing asthma exacerbations and lung damage. If control has not been established, then appropriate measures should be taken to do so. The patient's adherence to the medical regimen, proper technique for using inhaler devices, avoiding environmental triggers when possible, and identifying and treating any comorbidities that may destabilize asthma are all important [1], as is being aware of the other factors that impact high-risk inner-city asthmatics in particular.

The NHLBI/NAEPP Guidelines state specifically that one of the primary charges in managing asthma is to ensure that "all people who have asthma, particularly those at high risk, receive quality asthma care" [1]. This is easier said than done, but this charge can almost always be accomplished if asthma management is approached in a thoughtful manner. It is my opinion that preventing asthma exacerbations, particularly in high-risk asthmatics, should be the primary measure of effectiveness for all asthma management. At Advocate Health Care, tracking the frequency and severity of exacerbations in our asthma patient population is the primary outcomes metric that we use to monitor asthma morbidity and to help decrease resource utilization.

What Characterizes High-Risk Asthma?

High-risk asthma refers to those patients who are more likely to suffer high morbidity and death. Simply put, they need special attention. High-risk asthma patients are not all alike. They include not only those who have demonstrated a rocky clinical course with major life-threatening exacerbations, but also those who require high doses of inhaled or systemic corticosteroids in order to decrease the frequency of exacerbations. Some high-risk asthmatics find it difficult to avoid environmental asthma triggers, and some of have intense lung inflammation that requires daily systemic corticosteroid to attenuate their airways instability, even while they also continue the best maintenance medications available for long-term control.

High-risk asthma patients are readily identifiable (Fig. 18.4) [1].

Asthma History

Previous severe exacerbations (e.g. intubation or ICU admission for asthma)
Two or more hospitalizations for asthma in the past year
Three or more ED visits for asthma in the past year
Hospitalization or ED visit for asthma in the past month
Using >2 canisters of SABA per month
Difficulty perceiving asthma symptoms or severity of exacerbations
Other risk factors: lack of a written asthma action plan, sensitivity to *Alternaria*

Social History

Low socioeconomic status or inner-city residence
Illicit drug use
Major psychosocial problems

Comorbidities

Cardiovascular disease
Other chronic lung disease
Chronic psychiatric disease

Fig. 18.4 Risk factors for death from asthma

Such patients are found in all ethnic groups and in all socioeconomic strata, but are especially common among African–American children, African–American women, and Puerto Ricans. Others include obese women with adult-onset asthma, especially if they have nasal/sinus polyposis and an idiosyncratic reaction to aspirin and other nonsteroidal anti-inflammatory drugs, and also highly allergic asthmatics. Special measures must be taken to decrease the statistical probability of asthma attacks in these populations with special phenotypes. Aggressive treatment with inhaled corticosteroid (ICS) and/or combination therapy, avoidance of offending drugs, and control of environmental triggers are essential in decreasing these patients likelihood of experiencing premature asthma death and severe asthma exacerbations, especially if they have other risk factors for death from asthma [1].

All high-risk asthma is not the same as severe asthma. Certain demographic features automatically qualify patients as having high-risk asthma no matter how severe their disease appears to be clinically. Because national statistics show that African–American women and Puerto Ricans have the highest mortality due to asthma among all ethnic groups [9], we consider all African–American women with asthma to be very high-risk.

All patients with very poorly controlled asthma do not necessarily have severe asthma either. Some of them are simply nonadherent to their asthma medical regimen, while others are regularly exposed to asthma triggers that drive their asthma. Upon convincing these patients to adhere to treatment and extricating them from such environments, they tend to do much better. On the other hand, it is apparent that individuals with severe asthma require high-intensity asthma treatment. This group of patients includes some individuals with very poorly controlled asthma, some who can only achieve and maintain well-controlled asthma status while taking high-intensity asthma treatment, and others with frequent asthma exacerbations despite high-intensity treatment.

How Will High-Risk Asthma Be Defined in the Future?

Unfortunately, assessing current asthma control in response to various treatments – a trial and error process – is not always sufficient to produce optimal management decisions and outcomes. Ideally, we would also like to know the patient's underlying genetic and genomic characteristics and their clinical phenotype up front to personalize their treatments. This knowledge will become increasingly important as asthma therapies are developed to target specific components of the complex inflammatory response. Measuring individual patient's pathophysiological disease markers may then provide information about their future risks and predict their best treatments, making better sense out of the clinical variation that we can only observe at present. The morbidity and mortality of asthma will be impacted positively as our understandings of its underlying causes improve. Ultimately, the clinical expression of the syndrome we call asthma must be assessed and interpreted within the context of its multiple phenotypes, and fully appreciating the influence of socioeconomic status, race, and the clinical environment [10]. Hopefully, that time will come soon.

Special Considerations

The glucocorticoid-insensitive patient: Responsiveness to corticosteroids is a glaring example of the variation seen in asthma management with medicines and environmental manipulations. While the majority of patients with chronic persistent asthma respond to corticosteroid therapy, this treatment has little or no therapeutic effect for a small subgroup of patients [11]. Some of these individuals respond only to extremely high dosages; others are entirely unresponsive. Numerous factors may contribute, but in my clinical experience, the leading reason is the patient's suboptimal adherence to the treatment prescribed. Recognizing these difficult-to-treat patients is important, because they account for up to 50% of the economic burden of asthma disease management [12].

The recalcitrant asthmatic: Some of these severe asthmatics are not controlled in spite of the highest levels of recommended treatments. In others, control can only be achieved and maintained with the highest levels of recommended treatments [7, 13]. Some of these patients have what has been referred to as "corticosteroid-dependent asthma" because their control deteriorates whenever their maintenance of corticosteroid dose is reduced. Unfortunately, there are no validated tests to measure corticosteroid sensitivity, but some clinical studies show that obesity and tobacco smoke may contribute to decreased corticosteroid responsiveness [4, 7, 8].

Anticipatory Asthma Care: A Paradigm for the Outpatient Management of High-risk Urban Asthmatics

The complexities of asthma that I have described, its documented underdiagnosis and undertreatment, and its high direct and indirect costs mandate new approaches to asthma management. At Advocate Health Care, a large managed care organization in and near Chicago, we have developed a system-based project for several thousand high-risk asthma patients. We have acknowledged that urban patients' asthma has a heightened potential for poor outcomes, in part because subpopulations in urban America tend to experience asthma in its most severe form, in part because environmental variables increase their burden of asthma, and because the urban environment impacts chronic disease outcomes in general [14]. Within our population, perceptual barriers must frequently be addressed as well. As one example, an asthma exacerbation is frequently viewed "an event" instead of the end result of an uncontrolled chronic inflammatory airways disease [15].

Multiple studies show that systemwide interventions result in better health outcomes than provider-dependent strategies for large populations of asthma patients [16, 17]. In high-risk inner-city patients, these have ranged from the use of "breathmobiles", pioneered by Jones and his colleagues [18], to our Anticipatory Asthma Care (AAC) program (Fig. 18.5) [10].

At Advocate Health Care, the goal of, and responsibility for improving asthma outcomes is shared by the entire system, not left to the clinicians alone. We use an

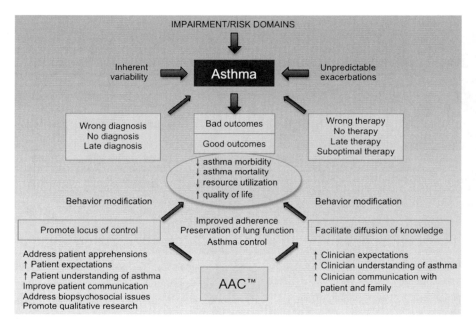

Fig. 18.5 Anticipatory asthma care (AAC) Program; adapted from reference 19

interdisciplinary, multidimensional approach to achieve buy-in by all staff, our primary care physicians, and our asthma specialists. Physician champions and asthma case managers were actively involved in the initial program design, and continue to contribute to its improvement. Our system-based interventions include standardized treatment protocols, standardized asthma action/treatment plans, and an asthma registry of high-risk patients based on both their prior resource utilization and our ongoing assessment of their risk and disease control. The NHLBI guidelines are used to assess asthma severity and control. The ACC paradigm is used to identify high-risk patients. Each patient's level of asthma control and risk status are then monitored over time.

Ongoing physician and nursing education focuses on establishing an early diagnosis. Primary care providers are strongly encouraged to make early referrals of high-risk asthmatics to our asthma specialists to facilitate comprehensive coordinated care, and to identify and modify disease management barriers. Quarterly medical record audits are used to generate a feedback report to primary care physicians, to improve asthma management, and to close gaps in care.

At Advocate Health Care, *"anticipating the worst-case scenario but planning for the best-case scenario"* has had a tremendous impact on our managing high-risk asthmatics. We have moved our clinicians away from "usual asthma care" to the "Anticipatory Asthma Care (AAC)" paradigm (Table 18.1) [19]. Case-based management and problem-based learning have been the primary methods used to achieve this transformation.

Table 18.1 Anticipatory asthma care (AAC) Paradigm: improving asthma outcomes, adapted from [10]

Usual Asthma Care	Anticipatory Asthma Care
No emphasis on "patient profiling"	Strong emphasis on "patient profiling"
Little emphasis on anticipating and predicting patient's adherence to the medical regimen	Strong emphasis on anticipating and predicting the patient's adherence to the medical regimen
Little emphasis on the patient's level of education	Strong emphasis on the patient's level of education
Passive interest in the patient's socioeconomic status	High interest in the patient's socioeconomic status
Passive interest in ascertaining the patient's belief system	High interest in ascertaining the patient's belief system (e.g., exploring the patient's locus of control; attempting behavior modification whenever necessary)
Little emphasis in short- and long-term medication side effects	Strong emphasis on short- and long-term side effects
Little emphasis on the patient's micro- and macro-environments and their respective impacts	Strong emphasis on the patient's micro- and macro-environments and their respective impacts
Little emphasis on spriometry and asthma action plans	Strong emphasis on spriometry and asthma action plans
Little reflection on the long-term ramifications of poorly controlled asthma and its potential complications, especially as they relate to comorbidities	Insightful reflection on the long-term ramifications of poorly controlled asthma and its potential complications, especially as they relate to comorbidities
Clinician adopts a "reactive" mindset, readily accepting a certain level of asthma disability	Clinician adopts a "proactive" mindset, and is intolerant of any asthma disability except in rare cases
Clinician is frequently caught "off guard" when the patient's clinical course and disposition change	Clinician anticipates and foresees unannounced changes in the patient's clinical course and anticipates the patient's needs
Clinician rarely anticipates the worst-case scenario	Clinician continually anticipates the worst-case scenario, but plans for the best-case scenario by always thinking "What can go wrong?"

Advocate Health Care achieved a fundamental behavior modification in re-allocating its resources to achieve more successful asthma disease management. In particular, we hired and reassigned nurses as full-time asthma disease managers. Previously, our case managers had been assigned patients with multiple diseases, including only those asthmatics with repeated hospital admissions or visits to the Emergency Department or Urgent Care facilities. They lacked formal training in asthma care and asthma patient education. With AAC, the objective shifted from reactive care of high-utilizing individuals to proactive management of our high-risk asthma population, and our asthma nurse managers were educated about the disease, its clinical management, and patient education methods.

The nurse managers' responsibility now includes updating our high-risk asthma registry every week. High-risk asthmatics are not only identified by reviewing

Urgent Care and Emergency Department visits and hospitalizations, but also by identifying those patients with adherence problems, psychosocial issues, and financial barriers to purchasing their asthma medicines. All our staff participate in identifying these high-risk patients – the case managers themselves, our primary care and emergency department providers, and our asthma specialists.

Our asthma case management includes three types of interactions between the case managers and the asthma patients: telephone encounters, office visits, and home site visits. The latter are used for asthmatics suspected of having environmental triggers that contribute to their asthma morbidity. A standardized asthma curriculum based on the NHLBI asthma guidelines is used for teaching high-risk asthmatics self-management skills and environmental control measures. A supply-stocking program ensures onsite availability of spacers, peak flow meters, and nebulizers for selected patients.

We have applied the NHLBI asthma guidelines uniformly throughout our asthma population. Our primary focus is to establish an internal locus of control for the patient. A partnership between the patient and the clinician is encouraged to facilitate early diagnosis, education, and optimal treatment. Consistent evidence-based asthma education is provided to both our clinicians and patients about the inflammatory nature of asthma, adherence to the medical regimen during periods of asthma stability and during exacerbations, and environmental control measures.

Advocate Health monitors our ACC results continuously. A multidisciplinary asthma disease management study showed success in many areas, but not all [16]. Documentation of asthma diagnosis and patient education has improved. Emergency department visits and hospitalizations have been reduced substantially. We have reduced asthma exacerbations, achieved lower morbidity and mortality rates, improved quality of life for patients and their families, reduced asthma resource utilization, and hopefully, have reduced premature loss of lung function in adults, and prevented decline in lung growth in children. In contrast, no improvements have been seen in peak flow meter ownership/use, smoking cessation advice, or influenza vaccination.

Conclusions

Managing and controlling asthma is challenging and complex, especially for those patients with high-risk disease. Our AAC paradigm at Advocate Health Care provides an example of system-based, interdisciplinary chronic disease management that has improved outcomes and costs consistent with the National Heart, Lung, and Blood Institute (NHLBI)/National Asthma Education Prevention Program (NAEPP) "Guidelines for the Diagnosis and Management of Asthma." We believe that the AAC paradigm can be adapted to a variety of clinical settings to improve the care high-risk asthma patients.

Editor's Comments: Michael Foggs is every allergist's go-to guy for best asthma care. He begins by convincing us that asthma management is a dizzying challenge, especially in urban high-risk patient populations. He then tells us how his system has applied treatment guidelines and system-based care principles to standardize population care without losing track of the individual patient. Once again, we are told that disease-specific nurse managers for high-risk patients are critical to overcoming the barriers to achieving high performance. Like the Marian CHF program, they have extended their services into their patients' homes. The evolution of risk-definition and measurement over time in his field is intriguing, and like other chronic diseases, genetic and genomic research offers an even brighter future. JTH

References

1. National Heart, Lung, and Blood Institute, National Asthma Education and Prevention Program. Expert Panel Report 3. *Guidelines for the Diagnosis and Management of Asthma.* Full report 2007. Bethesda MD: U.S. Department of Health and Human Services, 2007; NIH publication no. 07-4051.
2. Singh AM, Busse WW. Asthma exacerbations – 2: Aetiology. Thorax. 2006;61(9):809–16.
3. Moore WC, Meyers DA, Wenzel SE, et al. Identification of asthma phenotypes using cluster analysis in the Severe Asthma Research Program. Am J Respir Crit Care Med. 2010;181(4): 315–23.
4. Quinn K, Shalowitz MU, Berry CA, et al. Racial and ethnic disparities in diagnosed and possible undiagnosed asthma among public-school children in Chicago. Am J Public Health. 2006;96(9):1599–603.
5. Woolf SH, Grol R, Hutchinsonn A, et al. Potential benefits, limitations, and harms of clinical guidelines. Br Med J. 1999;318(7182):527–30.
6. Calhoun WJ, Sutton BB, Emmett A, et al. A variability in patients previously treated with ß-agonists alone. J Allergy Clin Immunol. 2003;112(6):1088–94.
7. Bousquet J, Mantzouranis E, Cruz AA, et al. Uniform definition of asthma severity, control, and exacerbations: document presented for the World Health Organization consultation on severe asthma. J Allergy Clin Immunol. 2010;126(5):926–38.
8. Haahtela T, Jävinen M, Kava T, et al. Effects of reducing or discontinuing inhaled budesonide in patients with mild asthma. N Engl J Med. 1994;331(11):700–5.
9. Centers for Disease Control and Prevention. National Center for Health Statistics. National Vital Statistics Report. Deaths: Final Data for 1999–2006. Trends in asthma morbidity and mortality. American Lung Association, Epidemiology and Statistics Unit, Research and Program Services Division. February, 2010.
10. Foggs MB. Influence of socioeconomic status, race, and clinical environment on asthma care. Respir Digest. 2005;7(2):1–13.
11. Malmstrom K, Rodriguez-Gomez G, Guerra J, et al. Oral montelukast, inhaled beclomethasone, and placebo for chronic asthma: a randomized, controlled trial. Ann Int Med. 1999; 130(6):487–95.
12. Chung KF, Godard P, Adelroth E, et al. Difficult/therapy-resistant asthma: the need for an integrated approach to define clinical phenotypes, evaluate risk factors, understand pathophysiology and find novel therapies. ERS task force on difficult/therapy-resistant asthma. European Respiratory Society. Eur Respir J. 1999;13(5):1198–208.
13. Wenzel S. Severe asthma in adults. Am J Respir Crit Care Med. 2005;172(2):149–60.
14. Bach PP, Pham HH, Schrag D, et al. Primary care physicians who treat blacks and whites. N Engl J Med. 2004;351(6):575–84.
15. Halm EA, Mora P, Leventhal H. No symptoms, no asthma: the acute episodic disease belief is associated with poor asthma self-management among inner-city adults with persistent asthma. Chest. 2006;129(3):573–80.

16. Patel PH, Welsh C, Foggs MB. Improved asthma outcomes using a coordinated care approach in a large medical group. Disease Manage. 2004;7(2):102–11.
17. Evans R, LeBailly S, Gordon KK, et al. Restructuring asthma care in a hospital setting to improve outcomes. Chest. 1999;116(4 Suppl 1):210S–6S.
18. Jones CA, Clement LT, Harley-Lopez J, et al. The Breathmobile program: structure, implementation, and evolution of a large-scale urban pediatric asthma disease management program. Disease Manage. 2005;8(4):205–22.
19. Foggs MB. Guidelines management of asthma in a busy urban practice. Curr Opin Pulm Med. 2008;14(1):46–56.

Chapter 19
Cardiovascular Disease: Reducing Risk Factors

Richard D. Lueker and Beth A. McCormick

Keywords New heart • Cardiac rehabilitation • Cardiovascular disease • Risk factors • Exercise • Comprehensive • Telehealth • Referral

Ezekiel 36:26 "I will give you a new heart, and put a new spirit within you."

The Beginning of New Heart

New Heart was born some 35 years ago in 1975, a time of strife and anxiety for the Lueker family – and of a miraculous encounter that changed our lives. My son Steve had been quite sick for months. Events peaked one night when I discovered lymph node swelling under his arms, in his neck, and in his groin area. He was crying in bed. I tried to comfort him as I examined him, but I was shocked and frightened by what I had found. He had been to the pediatrician repeatedly for his symptoms of swelling and pain of the elbow and then ankle. Laboratory tests had not been conclusive except for moderate anemia. I finally settled him down and got him to sleep. For hours, I walked the streets anxious and fearful. What was going on? I was in tears and cried out to the Lord: "Help me, please."

Two days later I received a call from Paul. "I know you haven't met me, but I had a nice visit with your mother about a year ago. She told me that if I ever got to Albuquerque, I should give you a call." I remembered my mother telling me about this gentleman she met on the train and how his demeanor impressed her. I asked him to come over to the house, and when he did later that day, I blurted out all the worry, fear, and anxiety that had been bundled up inside of me.

R.D. Lueker, MD (✉) • B.A. McCormick, MS
New Heart Center for Wellness, Fitness, and Cardiac Rehabilitation,
Albuquerque, NM, USA
e-mail: lueker.newheart@gmail.com

J.T. Harrington and E.D. Newman (eds.), *Great Health Care: Making It Happen*,
DOI 10.1007/978-1-4614-1198-7_19, © Springer Science+Business Media, LLC 2012

> As I finished, he smiled and said: "Now I understand why
> I came to Albuquerque this weekend."
>
> Paul was a retired Presbyterian minister whose quiet
> demeanor was indeed comforting. He asked if he could pray
> for my son. Very calmly, quietly, he asked for Steve to be
> healed. The next day, I found Steve running down the street. I
> jumped out of the car and ran to grab him. I said, "Don't you
> know you're sick?" He pulled away and exclaimed, "Dad,
> I'm fine!"
>
> I had witnessed a miracle. Months of anxiety, fear, and
> uncertainty gone in a space of 24 h. As I ruminated about these
> events, I was left thinking… "What response do I make to this
> happening?" That response was the birth of New Heart.

Richard Leuker

Jefferson Junior High School, 1973

In 1969, after finishing my cardiology fellowship and year on faculty at the University of Colorado, I joined the faculty at the University of New Mexico School of Medicine. The heart surgical program migrated to a private hospital in town and pulled many of us along. I practiced cardiology; did heart catheterization and angiography. This was at the very beginning of angioplasty. We had many patients with heart disease, and pondered how to help them more than just with medications. Was there something else? I had read a story in *Time* magazine about an individual who was involved in a cardiac rehabilitation program in Cleveland and was now running 1 mile a day approximately 1 year after a heart attack. This was a stimulus to develop a program here in Albuquerque. The data regarding the benefits of such programs was nowhere near what it is today.

I partnered with an exercise physiologist, Dr. Hemming Atterbom, and Dr. John Gustafson from the University of New Mexico physical education department. I also enlisted nurses and technicians from the nearby hospital to join us in the endeavor. We rented space at Jefferson Junior High School three evenings a week, and gathered several patients from my own and other cardiology practices. We started in December 1973. Participants walked around the gym. We had classes on heart disease. As folks became stronger they would go outside and run on the track. During the winter we put up lights on the fence so that our participants could jog around the parking lot. We did not do a walk test or any other formal assessment. The only medical information that we had on each patient was that provided by his or her primary care physician or cardiologist. That was the beginning.

Over subsequent years, the program grew dramatically, and today we are a non-profit 501(c)3 organization in a 12,000 square-foot facility ideal for teaching reha-bilitation and prevention, a gift from a prominent businessman who went through our program and later endowed us with over $3 million. It has been exciting over the years to see how the vision has expanded as the knowledge and benefits of cardiac rehabilitation have been validated.

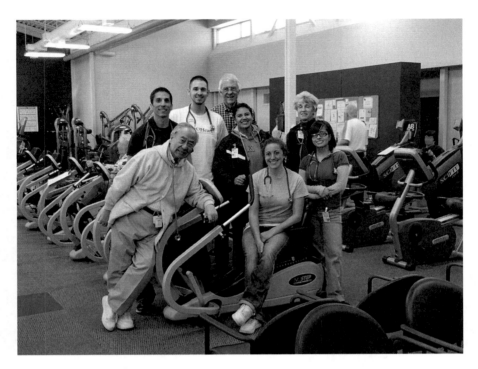

Fig. 19.1 The New Heart team picture shows author Dick Lueker, "the tall guy with white hair (blond according to him!) in the back", in the words of coauthor Beth McCormick, who is behind the camera, and refused to disclose her own hair color

Current Program

Clinical Visits. Patients are referred from surrounding hospitals and cardiac clinics. They have all had coronary disease, a heart attack, angioplasty, coronary bypass surgery or, on occasion, valve repair or replacement. The initial visit is very comprehensive, beginning with a treadmill test and electrocardiogram to determine a safe heart rate for exercise, as part of their exercise prescription. It also includes heart rate, blood pressure, number of minutes on the treadmill, height, weight, waist circumference, a body mass index, a dietary score, anxiety and depression scores, and their level of physical activity over the past week in kilocalories per week and metabolic hours per week. Immediately after the treadmill test, each patient visits with one of our physicians for 30 min to discuss these assessments, the risk factors they represent, and the goals for the individual's cardiac rehabilitation program. During a typical 12-week program, progress in these metrics is assessed at 4, 8, and 12 weeks (Fig. 19.1).

Patients visit at least once with our dietitian, who assists them in establishing a healthy eating program. Our sizeable population of individuals with diabetes is provided specific dietary programs. A behavioral health specialist meets with patients at 2 and 10 weeks to discuss any barriers to behavior change and important emotional issues that might be related to their heart disease or rehabilitation process.

Finally, for those individuals who have a strong family history of heart disease, a history of recurrent cardiac events, or a diagnosis of coronary disease at a young age, "advanced lipid testing" and evaluation are strongly recommended. This provides us with very meaningful data regarding the size and number of lipid particles, which assists in prescribing a precise medication program to alter their abnormal lipids. An abnormal cholesterol particle number predicts more severe disease or more recurrent problems. Identifying these people and modifying their cholesterol medications reduces their ongoing risk.

> A scientist presented to New Heart after a heart attack some 18 years ago. He was 47 years of age, very slender, fit, and active as a soccer coach and referee. "How can this be happening to me," he cried. I had no good answers. Five years later, he returned after another myocardial infarction. The science of lipid testing and treatment had advanced in the meantime, and we identified his cholesterol particle abnormality, which responded to additional medical therapy. He has now been free of any recurrent cardiac events for 13 years.

Exercise Protocols on the Floor. Individuals with coronary disease need to have ECG monitoring during exercise to detect any abnormal rhythms. Initially, patients are given instructions for applying electrodes and a telemetry monitor, which allows staff to evaluate their rhythms while they exercise. Participants are given instructions in using exercise equipment, which include treadmills, stationary bikes, NuStep machines, and a variety of others designed to increase aerobic capacity, and weight-training machines are available to improve muscular strength.

An exercise prescription is more difficult than other prescriptions that physicians might provide because every person is unique: different age, different body strength, and habitus. During the treadmill test, the patient walks until he or she indicates the level of exercise is moderately difficult. The heart rate at that time is used to calculate an exercise heart rate, which is approximately 20% less than the heart rate of peak exercise. The ECG is also reviewed to exclude any problems at that moment.

As the patient's minutes of exercise increase over the next few weeks, the exercise heart rate may be increased. Frequently, patients show considerable increases in their exercise time. The goal is at least 60 min of exercise three times a week in the New Heart gym, with additional walking at home on two other days. Several past research studies, including the Harvard Alumni Study and the Heidelberg Study, have shown reduced mortality and morbidity in those who achieved over 2,000 kcal of exercise weekly [1, 2].

Weight training is very important for humans as they age, even for persons in their 80s or 90s. It is particularly important for the legs, as it reduces the risk of falls and allows a person to walk at lower levels of exertion or energy expenditure.

Outcomes. Subjectively, the majority of participants indicate a significant improvement in their overall strength and energy. Usually I ask, "Are you a nickel, or a quarter, or 50 cents better?" It is not unusual for a participant 8 weeks into the program to state, "I am a dollar better." I ask, "You mean 100% better?" and receive the affirmative reply. Recent evidence shows a dramatic benefit for those who complete the entire cardiac rehabilitation program. In a 2010 report in *Circulation*, Hammill and colleagues showed that among 30,161 Medicare beneficiaries who qualified for and attended at least one cardiac rehabilitation session, those who had attended all 36 had a 47% lower risk of death and a 31% lower risk of myocardial infarction after 4 years, when compared with those who attended only one session [3]. One of our primary goals, therefore, is to retain participants through a full 36 exercise sessions.

At 12 weeks, as patients complete the initial program, their amount of exercise expressed in energy expenditure increases over 300% from baseline on average. We often see significant improvements in blood pressure (both systolic and diastolic), such that some participants have lowered the dose of medication or discontinued medication entirely. Exercise and improved fitness lead to such changes more often than we had thought possible in the past.

Improvements in cholesterol (both LDL and HDL) levels are common. This is important because significant LDL cholesterol reduction (to 70 mg/dL) may cause very substantial regression of cholesterol plaque within 24 months [4]. During the 12-week program, stress scores usually fall considerably, and depression and anxiety scores may also improve (Figs. 19.2 and 19.3).

Long-Term Goals

We start people on the road to recovery, but the 12 weeks of cardiac rehabilitation is just the warm-up period. The really important part is what happens afterward. We keep about 60% of individuals in the program through 12 weeks. Of these, about 50% move into our Preventing Heart Disease (PHD) maintenance program and continue exercising at New Heart. These are invariably our biggest success stories. These people have accepted not only the value of cardiac rehab, but also the value of being at New Heart, where there is a positive, encouraging culture. We do not put undue pressure on anyone, but also do not allow any slacking off. For the 50% who do not stay at New Heart, we try to schedule 6-month and annual follow-ups during which we conduct a walk test and evaluate current health status and healthy activities. This is a less than ideal way of helping individuals maintain improvements over time, and many individuals are lost to follow-up.

We find that education is a critical part of the successes we see in our patients. Our clinical staff all endeavor to provide individualized instruction and advice that reinforces the strengths of each individual. We also employ Motivational Interviewing techniques to help individuals overcome ambivalence toward change, identify what they value most, and make the choices that will help them achieve their own goals [5].

Patient Stories

We can anticipate fairly predictable results in patients who follow a prescribed cardiac rehabilitation program, complete all 36 exercise sessions, and continue some sort of exercise and nutrition routine after graduating from our program. However,

Progress Report

New♡Heart
Center for Wellness, Exercise and Cardiac Rehabilitation

Patient		DOB				
Physiological Variables						
Assessment Date		9/3/02	10/25/02	12/6/02	4/11/03	8/1/03
Assessment						Yearly
Resting Heart Rate		65	67	63	66	65
Exercising Target HR		110-120		110-120	110-120	110-120
Resting SBP		94	108	118	112	94
Resting DBP		70	64	50	82	70
METs at Moderate Intensity		4.13		8.03	9.45	8.03
Limited Walk Test (METs)		4.13		7.06	10.13	8.43
Pre CBG						na
Post CBG						na
Body Composition	**Desirable**					
Weight		164.5	156	152	148	150
Body Mass Index	<25	29	27	27	26	26
Waist Circumference	m<40/f<35	35	33	32	30.5	33
Lifestyle-Related Measures	**Desirable**					
Fat Intake Score	Low	High	Low	Low	Low	Low
Fruit/Veg Intake Score	High	Mod.	High	High	High	Low
Anxiety Score	<8					
Depression Score	<8					
Exercise kcal / week		171	1352	1984	2010	1995
Exercise MET-hrs/wk	>12	2.2	18.2	27.3	28.2	27.7
Perceived Stress Score	Low	High	Mod.	Low	Low	Low
Cigarettes per day	0	0	0	0	0	0
Medication Compliance (%)	100	100	100	100	100	100

Comments   10/25/02-Pt. c/o having cold hands and feet all the time. CM

New Heart Inc. · 601 Lomas Blvd NE · Albuquerque, NM 87102 · 505.881.8195

Fig. 19.2 Individual patient progress report

some individuals go above and beyond our greatest expectations. They embrace the new opportunities given to them by the recovery process, and they soar to new heights of endeavor and accomplishment. Here are a few success stories (Fig. 19.4):

Doyle Wise had a family history of cardiac disease. His father had experienced a heart attack and two brothers had undergone bypass surgery in the past. Though he had good dietary habits, Doyle did not exercise regularly and had high cholesterol. In 2003, at age 66, he suffered a heart attack and subsequently underwent quadruple

Table 1. New Heart Cardiac Rehabilitation Program Graduate Demographics (2007, 2008 and 2009 Cummulative Outcomes Summary).

Parameter	N	Percent (%)	Age *
Patients – Overall	384	100.00%	66.70±10.86
Female	115	29.95%	68.32±10.80
Male	269	70.05%	66.00±10.84
Diabetes	106	27.60%	67.28±11.04

* Values are means±standard deviation.

Table 2. New Heart Cardiac Rehabilitation Program Graduate, Outcome Data (2007, 2008 and 2009 Cummulative Outcomes Summary).

Outcome variable	Baseline	12-week	% change
Stress score (goal<14)	12.61 ± 6.67	10.32 ± 6.44	**-18.14%**
Fat intake score (goal<8)	11.09 ± 5.90	9.32 ± 5.22	**-15.97%**
Energy expenditure (kcal/wk) (goal >1000, >1500, >2200)	273.51 ± 563.73	1218.34 ± 775.77	**345.45%**
METs attained on Submax Walking Test (goal>5, >8, >10)	4.03 ± 1.86	5.74 ± 2.45	**42.54%**
Systolic BP (goal <120mmHg)	119.78 ± 15.60	117.80 ± 14.47	**-1.65%**
Diastolic BP (goal <80mmHg)	73.40 ± 9.65	70.95 ± 8.76	**-3.34%**
Total cholesterol (mg/dL) (goal <200, <150) *185/384=48.18%	161.39 ± 44.14	144.54 ± 32.39	**-10.44%**
HDL (mg/dL) >40, >60 *186/384=48.44%	40.45 ± 12.76	43.84 ± 13 03	**8.38%**
Female (goal HDL >50, >60)	46.55 ± 13.91	51.34 ± 14 74	**10.30%**
Male (goal HDL >40, >60)	38.00 ± 11.43	40.83 ± 10.96	**7.44%**
LDL (mg/dL) (goal <100, <70) *179/384=46.61%	92.60 ± 37.66	77.13 ± 27.04	**-16.71%**
Advanced Lipid Testing	67 (17.45%) Tested/384 Total	48 (71.64%)= B Pattern/67 tested	19 (28.36%)= A Pattern/67 tested
Triglycerides (goal <150mg/dL) *183/384=47.66%	153.66 ± 118.84	124.78 ± 73.69	**-18.79%**
Body mass index (kg/m²) (goal <30, <25)	28.08 ± 5.03	28.03 ± 5.01	**-0.16%**
Waist Circumference (inches)	39.37 ± 5.48	38.96 ± 5.03	**-1.03%**
Female Circ (goal <35)	37.21 ± 6.65	36.71 ± 5.69	**-1.36%**
Male Circ (goal ≤40)	40.30 ± 4.61	39.94 ± 4.39	**-0.90%**
New Heart Graduates with DIABETES (106)			
Fasting Blood Glucose (mg/dL) (goal <126, <110, <100) *14/106=13.21%	122.50 ± 41.49	114.21 ± 34.92	**-6.76%**
Hemoglobin A1c, (%), (goal<7.0, <6.2) *26/106=24.53%	7.37± 1.72	6.83 ± 1.20	**-0.53%**
Values are Mean ± standard deviation.			revisited 03/03/2010gr

Goals are based on ACSM's Resource Manual for Guidelines for Exercise Testing and Prescription, 5th Ed

*only patients with both pre and post labs were included in average and standard deviation calculations

Fig. 19.3 Aggregate patient outcomes 2006–2009

bypass. After coming to New Heart, Doyle began a regular exercise regimen, which he continues to this day. He has been much more active and energetic since the bypass. At age 71, Doyle and a group of friends undertook a 14-day walk across England. Traveling more than 200 miles through the lake country from the Irish Sea

Fig. 19.4 Doyle Wise at the
end of his journey across
England

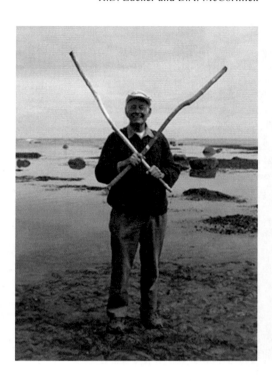

to the North Sea, Doyle commented "The British don't know what a switchback is. We would come to a hill and just go straight up."

With the support of his wife, the encouragement of his physicians, and proper training, Doyle made the trip without anxiety or incident. He stresses the importance of cardiac rehab referrals for patients undergoing heart surgery. Doyle's brother, who had no rehab, needs to rest every hour or so. Doyle considers him an invalid. In addition to rehab, Doyle says it is important to have social support from family and friends.

All his life, Rudy Matalucci had been an active person, enjoying racket sports, hiking and cross-country skiing. Though he developed dyslipidemia and hypothyroidism at age 45, Rudy continued to be active. In March 2007, at age 69, Rudy was hospitalized with bowel and chest pain diagnosed as an acute coronary syndrome. After having two stents placed, Rudy was referred to New Heart for cardiac rehabilitation (Fig. 19.5).

In the hospital, Rudy had been concerned that he would not be able to continue his physical activities, but doctors assured him that, if he continued exercising, he would be able to maintain his active retirement. After only 4 months at New Heart, Rudy took his first post-event hiking trip, a 5-day event in central Idaho reaching elevations of 11,000 ft. Since then, he has made similar expeditions in Chama, NM; Leadville, CO; the Sierra Nevada in California; and the Wind River Wilderness in Wyoming. Through hard work, constant training, optimism, support from family and friends, willpower, and by living in the moment through the spirit, Rudy has hardly missed a beat in his goal to live a vigorous and active life.

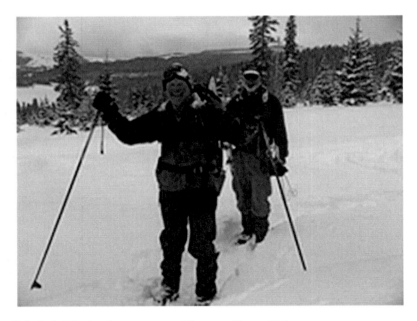

Fig. 19.5 Rudy Matalucci cross-country skiing near Chama, NM

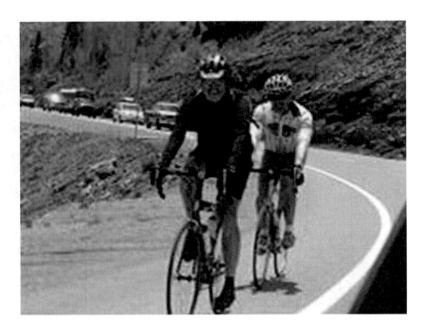

Fig. 19.6 Durand Smith on the iron horse trail

In June 2005, at the age of 57, Durand Smith had a fainting spell in his back yard. When he awoke with chest pain and nausea and vomiting, he went to the emergency room. Durand was diagnosed with an inferior wall myocardial infarction. While in the emergency room, Durand suffered a cardiac arrest, but was successfully resuscitated. After having one stent placed emergently and being put on an intra-aortic balloon pump pending surgery, Durand underwent triple bypass the following day. Though his postoperative recovery was uneventful, Durand suffered from extreme fatigue. He recalls having to sit down several times during his short initial tour of New Heart. He identifies some of the problems that contributed to his heart disease as a family history of early heart disease (his father, at age 45), a cholesterol level of 315 mg/dL, a highly stressful job where he managed 125 people and put in 70–80 h per week as a physicist for a major aerospace company, and a lack of exercise (Fig. 19.6).

After his cardiac event, Durand decided to make a major life change for his health. Now, he is in a company of ten people, is much more in touch with the technical aspects of his work, and is at New Heart by 3 p.m. every day to work out. Durand's anchor that guided him toward his current level of fitness was the Iron Horse Bicycle Classic, a 45-mile trek from Durango to Silverton, CO that goes through two 11,000 foot passes on the way. Not satisfied with building up to an hour of exercise per day, Durand began training for the race and, less than a year after being in cardiac arrest in his back yard, he accomplished his goal and completed the Iron Horse race in 9½ h. Durand says he could not have done what he did going to just any health club. He describes the atmosphere at New Heart as very positive, and said he became motivated to come back from his event and discover what his limits are.

Though these stories make it sound like rehabilitation is a walk in the park, it is not. It is a struggle for everyone. But it is a personal struggle that is different for each individual. Most patients do not know what to expect and many are frightened, depressed and anxious. One of the most powerful salves for this kind of tension is to encourage patients to share their personal stories with other patients.

> I remember one day when I was teaching a class to new cardiac rehab patients. I brought along a patient who had already completed the rehab process and asked him to share a little bit about his experience. As he began to speak, the patients in class asked him question after question. At first I thought, wait a minute, I'm the doctor, I'm supposed to be teaching this class. Then I realized the best thing I could do was sit down, shut up, and let this man share the power of his accomplishment with those who had yet to reach the other side of the journey. I had never been down the road these patients were facing and I could not offer them the same kind of reassurance and knowledge as the man who had already succeeded in the rehab process. It is wise to remember that, as physicians, we do not necessarily know the whole story. Let others share what they know. It may light the way for many more.

Program Structure

Over the past 37 years, New Heart has had many different looks and locations. Our current incarnation is a product of experience, mistakes, blessings, and good advice.

Staff. The core of our staff is a group of exercise physiologists and exercise technicians, most of whom have trained in the University of New Mexico's (UNM) esteemed exercise science program. The clinical staff includes a licensed dietitian/diabetes educator, a behavioral health specialist (a graduate student mentored by a UNM professor in health psychology), two internists, and a cardiologist. Two to three interns from the exercise science program supplement the exercise staff each semester. The administrative staff includes a coordinator and a billing and reception staff of four individuals. The final, critical staff member is an educator/recruiter who visits patients at the Heart Hospital of New Mexico during their inpatient stays. This person educates all heart patients on the benefits of exercise and recommends entry into a cardiac rehabilitation program, either at New Heart or at another facility, for those who qualify for insurance reimbursement.

Affiliations. Unlike most cardiac rehabilitation programs in the U.S., New Heart is an independent, unaffiliated entity located in a freestanding facility, not a hospital. This allows us to maintain our identity, control the atmosphere in which our program takes place, and provide the type of care we determine, through experience and attention to the medical literature, to be the best possible. This has also allowed us to foster relationships with many different providers, and to establish contracts or agreements with many facilities and medical groups to provide cardiac rehabilitation and prevention services to their patients.

Growth. Over the years, the size of the staff has increased and decreased with the number of active members in our various programs. In addition, the hours of operation have changed from a few hours each evening to every day, to 8 h a day, 3 days a week – our current schedule. Each of our three physicians covers 1 day of rehab. Our two internists have other sources of income to meet their financial needs. As medical director, I cover one cardiac rehab day and receive income for one additional day of administrative duties. It may seem unreasonable to try to find physicians with the flexibility and alternative resources to accommodate this type of schedule, but we have not had difficulty in doing so. There are many physicians in transition periods of their lives, perhaps nearing retirement, who are looking for a slower-paced workday.

In addition to having between 60 and 70 individuals in the cardiac rehabilitation program at any given time, we also have about 600 individuals in our PHD maintenance program and about 300 in the Silver Sneakers program, a Medicare funded gym membership for seniors. We offer a variety of group fitness classes including yoga, tai chi, EnhanceFitness, and Silver Sneakers. In addition, we have grant-funded contracts with two different Indian Health Service clinics to provide exercise programs for their patients with diabetes. We also try to enrich people's experience at New Heart with occasional live music, monthly birthday parties, heart-healthy potlucks, and annual Christmas parties. We have endeavored to create a community that revolves around wellness.

From 2003 to 2008, we conducted a cardiac rehabilitation program via a telehealth connection to the Rehoboth McKinley Christian Hospital in Gallup, NM,

150 miles from Albuquerque. Through a face-to-face and voice-to-voice real-time connection, our physicians met with patients throughout their exercise program, which was overseen by a nurse and an exercise technician in the Gallup hospital. The outcomes for patients in this program were equivalent to those who undergo cardiac rehabilitation on site in Albuquerque.

Healthcare System. Over the years, New Heart has found a niche and established a sustaining pool of resources from which to receive patients. The University of New Mexico Hospital and another major healthcare provider each have their own cardiac rehabilitation programs. However, the other major healthcare provider for the city, as well as the independent Heart Hospital of New Mexico, and many cardiac clinics, refer almost exclusively to New Heart. So essentially, the three programs work in parallel and do not compete.

Despite our ample sources of referral, we have found that, regardless of the value that various providers put on cardiac rehabilitation and prevention services, they often forget to send their patients our way. Nationwide, only about 13% of individuals who qualify for cardiac rehabilitation actually receive the service. In New Mexico, the percentage is even lower, at about 8% [6]. This is partly due to patients declining services, but it is also often due to a failure of the referral system. The best means of combating this problem is to have an educator/recruiter in place in a hospital, as we do at the Heart Hospital of New Mexico. Another solution is to have cardiac rehabilitation as a standing order on discharge forms for cardiac surgical patients. Providing physician's offices with faxable referral forms also facilitates the process. Maintaining contact with physicians, discharge planners, and case managers is critical. It is also imperative that staff facilitate the referral process, making it as simple as possible. If it is difficult to access and use the services, providers will not come back.

It is also critical to respect other people's territories. Our physicians do not attempt to change medications or provide care that is rightly provided by another physician. We continually keep referring providers apprised of what we are doing with their patients, and seek out their advice when we believe attention is required. Perhaps most importantly, we make sure patients have a positive experience. Our former patients are often our biggest advocates, cheerleaders, and donors. They will see that more patients come our way. Finally, there is probably no substitute for being in practice a long time. Colleagues learn to trust you and will help you when they can.

Current Problems

Two primary problems plague the cardiac rehabilitation business: finances and referrals. Research has shown that cardiac rehab is reimbursed at about 75% of the cost of providing the service [7]. Without some form of supplement or subsidy, programs cannot survive. Our primary source of supplementation is a cardiac risk reduction and maintenance program. This self-pay program includes approximately 900 members and provides 30% of our total revenues. It is also critical that we maintain a 501(c)3 nonprofit status, which allows us to conduct regular fundraising activities and to actively seek donations.

Cardiac rehabilitation is currently only reimbursed for patients with a few very specific diagnoses, and for those with a relatively recent qualifying event (within the past 6 to 12 months). Many others could benefit from the intervention. Even among those who do qualify, many must pay hefty co-pays. At $50 per exercise session, plus office visits, some patients must pay more than $2000 out of pocket for cardiac rehab. We are evaluating the feasibility of creating a patient assistance fund, which would alleviate the burden for those with true financial need.

The referral problem is more complex, but may be more amendable to modification and improvement. Though there are many issues that lead to the poor participation rate identified earlier, a large part of the problem lies in the motivation and behavior arena. We are diligently searching for methods to motivate patients to see the need for cardiac rehab and to make the leap. Getting them in the door is half the battle. Transportation is another problem that is difficult to solve, particularly in a large, rural state such as New Mexico. In the past, we had a van that transported patients, but the size of our program and the liability and cost issues prevent us from providing this service today. There are various transportation resources provided by government and private entities, but they remain inadequate for the need and are cost prohibitive for some.

These challenges keep us thinking day and night about how to provide our services to more people, and how to shift the societal attitudes such that people readily perceive the benefits of cardiac rehab and are eager to participate. Given the continuing poor reports on the rise of obesity and diabetes in our country, we must continue to be vigilant and seek out new ways to stem the tide.

The Future

Evidence has continued to show more and more clearly over the past 30 or so years that cardiovascular disease is largely preventable, particularly if major risk factors are addressed. This evidence has opened doors to huge opportunities. Improving modifiable risk factors including diabetes, obesity, hypertension, dyslipidemia, sedentary lifestyle, and poor nutrition may allow a considerable positive shift in the risk of cardiovascular disease. We have begun to look at how we can impact these risk factors with the expertise and physical resources we have accumulated to treat heart disease. We are seeking accreditation to provide diabetes self-management education, a rigorously tested program that helps those with diabetes learn to control blood sugar and make long-term behavior changes that will slow the progression of the disease process and curb the development of complications. We also see a number of patients for lipid management, and we provide weight loss programs for those who are interested.

As we move more and more into prevention, we realize the need to reach out into the community, seek out those with cardiac risk factors, and attempt to change the environment in which these risk factors develop and thrive. Through grant funding, local business donations, and our own financial reserves, we are creating programs that attempt to change the nature of how we live within our own communities. In the end, regardless of whether we are treating patients after a cardiac event, or those at risk of heart disease, the basic prescription is the same. Exercise and nutrition are critical in the prevention of disease, and long-term behavior change is the ultimate goal. If we can facilitate this process, we have done our jobs well.

Editor's Comments: The New Heart Program began with secondary prevention of new cardiac events in those whose high future risks are defined by a sentinel event. Dick Leuker is viewed as a visionary in his field; he saw it early and has stayed the course. He and his team have maintained their initial focus, but have also addressed the broad array of cardiac risk factors through expanding primary and secondary prevention, and creating a holistic approach to encouraging patients to change their lives for the better. They have developed a strong culture of clinical measurement, and a broad range of motivational methods to increase patients' adherence. Their ongoing problems with identifying and engaging the at-risk population and with funding for services of demonstrated high value are widely shared across chronic disease management programs. JTH

References

1. Paffenbarger RS, Hyde RT, Wing AL, Hsieh CC. Physical activity, all-cause mortality, and longevity of college alumni. N Engl J Med. 1986;314(10):605–13.
2. Neibauer J, Hambrecht R, Velich T, et al. Attenuated progression of coronary artery disease after 6 years of multifactorial risk intervention. Circulation. 1997;96:2534–41.
3. Hammill BG, Curtis LH, Schulman KA, Whellan DJ. Relationship between cardiac rehabilitation and long-term risks of death and myocardial infarction among elderly Medicare beneficiaries. Circulation. 2010;121:63–70.
4. Nissen SE, Nicholls SJ, Sipahi I, et al. Effect of very high-intensity statin therapy on regression of coronary atherosclerosis. JAMA. 2006;295(13):1556–65.
5. Miller WR, Rollnick S. Motivational interviewing: preparing people for change. 2nd ed. New York, NY: The Guilford; 2002.
6. Suaya JA, Shepard DS, Normand ST, Ades PA, Prottas J, Stason WB. Use of cardiac rehabilitation by Medicare beneficiaries after myocardial infarction or coronary bypass surgery. Circulation. 2007;116:1653–62.
7. Lee JA, Shepard DS. Costs of cardiac rehabilitation and enhanced lifestyle modification programs. J Cardiopulm Rehabil. 2009;29(6):348–57.

Chapter 20
Obesity: The Elephant in the Room

**Karen Cooper, Philip Schauer, Stacy Brethauer,
and Sangeeta Kashyap**

Keywords Obesity • BMI • Bariatric and metabolic institute • Sleep apnea • Diabetes
• Bariatric surgery • Gastric bypass • Gastric banding • Outcomes

At 33 years old, William already weighed 300 lbs with a Body Mass Index of 46 when the sudden deaths of his fiancée and father triggered his using food as a coping mechanism, and he gained an additional 400 lbs over the next 3–4 years.

At 700 lbs, William suffered an injury to his knee. It buckled under him, he fell, was unable to get up, and lay on the floor at home for 4 days. By coincidence, a family member stopped by, and called for emergency medical services. By then, William had developed rhabdomyolysis – muscle damage with release of toxic muscle chemicals into the bloodstream, was in renal failure, and had severe edema. He spent 4 months recovering in the hospital. He was transferred to a specialized nursing home for further rehabilitation and inpatient weight management, where he lost 235 lbs over the next 2 years.

In 2009, he was then admitted to the Cleveland Clinic's Metabolic and Bariatric Institute for surgical weight management at a presurgical weight of 466 lbs. Within 1 year after surgery, he lost 114 additional pounds, and changed his lifestyle permanently. He now exercises daily, pays attention to calories consumed, uses behavioral techniques for coping when stressed, and is looking forward to returning to his hometown to reunite with his daughter and significant other.

Why wasn't William's morbid obesity addressed before it escalated? Do we health care providers, family members, and the general public lack the courage to address the obesity epidemic that is occurring before our eyes?

K. Cooper, DO (✉) • P. Schauer, MD • S. Brethauer, MD • S. Kashyap, MD
Bariatric and Metabolic Institute, The Cleveland Clinic, Cleveland, OH, USA
e-mail: cooperk2@ccf.org

J.T. Harrington and E.D. Newman (eds.), *Great Health Care: Making It Happen*,   187
DOI 10.1007/978-1-4614-1198-7_20, © Springer Science+Business Media, LLC 2012

Definition and Etiology

Obesity has become an important public health problem in industrialized countries throughout the world. Body Mass Index (BMI = weight (kg)/(height (m))^2) is the primary measurement used to categorize obese patients. (Table 20.1) Excess body weight (EBW) is defined as the amount of weight present in excess of Ideal Body Weight (IBW) (as determined by Metropolitan Life Tables). In 1991, the National Institutes of Health defined morbid obesity as a BMI of 35 kg/m^2 or greater with severe obesity-related comorbidity, or a BMI of 40 kg/m^2 or greater without comorbidity [1].

The development of obesity involves interactions between excessive intake, inefficient calorie utilization, reduced metabolic activity, a reduced thermogenic response to meals, and an abnormally high set point for body weight. The thermogenic response is the body's rate of heat loss in response to calorie intake, and the set point is the individual's self perception of their normal weight range. Genetic, environmental, and psychosocial factors all contribute to this problem.

Prevalence and Risk Factors

The prevalence of obesity in the United States has increased from 15% in 1980 to 32% in 2004 [2]. The prevalence of extreme obesity (BMI ≥40) is 2.8% in men and 6.9% in women. The prevalence of childhood and adolescent obesity has tripled since 1980, and currently, 17% of US children and adolescents are overweight. Obesity and morbid obesity affect women and minorities, particularly middle-aged Black and Hispanic women, more than white males. Recent studies have also determined that childhood weight influences adulthood weight. Being overweight during older childhood is highly predictive of adult obesity, especially if a parent is also obese. Being overweight during the adolescent years is an even greater predictor of adult obesity. However, in almost every age and ethnic group, the prevalence of overweight or obesity exceeds 50%.

Obesity is now the second leading predictor of preventable death after cigarette smoking in the United States despite expenditures of over $45 billion annually on weight loss products [3].

Table 20.1 Definitions of obesity

Category	BMI	% Over IBW
Underweight	<18.5	
Normal	18.5–24.9	
Overweight	25–29.9	
Obesity (Class 1)	30–34.9	>20%
Severe Obesity (Class 2)	35–39.9	>100%
(Class 3)	40–49.9	
Superobesity	>50	>250%

Pathophysiology and Natural History

Adipose tissue is located primarily in the subcutaneous tissue and abdominal cavity. In general, females are more likely to deposit fat in the peripheral tissues, and males in the abdomen. As obesity develops, the size and number of fat cells increase. As fat cells grow, they release increasing amounts of inflammatory cytokines and decreased amounts of adiponectin, a hormone that positively regulates the metabolism of fat and glucose. These chemical changes contribute to the proinflammatory state associated with obesity and have deleterious effects on lipid and glucose metabolism.

Obesity shortens the life span of those who suffer with it. The age-adjusted mortality rate of an individual with a BMI $\geq$40 kg/m^2 is double that of a normal weight individual [4]. A man in his twenties with a BMI over 45 kg/m^2 will have a 22% reduction of 13 years in life expectancy [5]. The majority of obesity-related deaths are due to complications of diabetes and cardiovascular disease. Worldwide, approximately 2.5 million deaths occur annually due to obesity-related comorbidities.

Signs, Symptoms, and Related Diseases

There are over 30 comorbid conditions associated with severe obesity. Insulin resistance and diabetes mellitus occur in 15–25% of obese patients. Increased abdominal fat raises the intra-abdominal pressure, contributing to gastroesophageal reflux, urinary stress incontinence, venous stasis disease, and abdominal hernias. Fatty deposits in the liver can progress to nonalcoholic steatohepatitis (NASH), and ultimately to liver failure. Excess weight can lead to debilitating back and joint diseases. The low-grade inflammatory state that is associated with morbid obesity contributes to vascular and coronary artery disease, and to clotting disorders seen commonly in these patients. Obese patients have impaired pulmonary function, particularly decreased lung capacity, and frequently suffer from asthma, obstructive sleep apnea, and obesity hypoventilation syndrome (Pickwickian syndrome). Other comorbidities include hypertension, dyslipidemia, and sex hormone dysfunction. Obesity is associated with an increased incidence of uterine, breast, ovarian, prostate, and colon cancer, and an excess of skin infections, urinary tract infections, migraine headaches, depression, and pseudotumor cerebri – a swelling of brain tissue.

Diagnosis and Evaluation of Comorbidities

The diagnosis of morbid obesity is established by determining the patient's Body Mass Index and the presence of any significant comorbid conditions. A thorough history, physical exam, and focused testing will uncover previously undiagnosed comorbidities in up to two-thirds of obese patients.

Table 20.2 ATP III criteria for metabolic syndrome. Three or more of the following

Central obesity	
Waist circumference in men	>102 cm
Waist circumference in women	>88 cm
Hypertriglyceridemia	≥150 mg/dl
Low HDL cholesterol	
Men	<40 mg/dl
Women	<50 mg/dl
High blood pressure	≥130/≥85 mm Hg
Fasting blood glucose	≥110 mg/dl

Cholesterol Education Program (NCEP) Expert Panel on Detection, Evaluation, and Treatment of High Blood Cholesterol in Adults (Adult Treatment Panel III) final report. (6), with permission

Visceral or central fat is more metabolically active than peripheral fat, and in excess, it more commonly leads to the Metabolic Syndrome defined in Table 20.2 [6], and consisting of Type 2 diabetes, dyslipidemia (elevated triglycerides and reduced HDL), high blood pressure, and an increased risk for atherosclerotic cardiovascular disease. The waist-to-hip ratio helps to identify patients with excess visceral adiposity. Women with waist-to-hip ratios of more than 0.8 and men with a ratio of more than 1.0 are considered to have excess central adiposity.

Obesity Management at the Cleveland Clinic

The Cleveland Clinic reorganized its obesity care into an interdisciplinary Bariatric and Metabolic Institute in 2005 to improve the continuum of care for obese patients who had previously been referred to our bariatric surgeons, or had received care in separate medical departments. Our professional team includes medical bariatricians, bariatric surgeons, dietitians, psychologists, clinical nurse specialists, and business staff. Our bariatric facilities provide one-stop shopping for obese patients and provide them their own space. Unique resources include spacious exam rooms, large furniture, and specialized scales and exam tables. A bariatric endoscopy suite allows procedures to be integrated with other care. Other medical services participate in evaluating and managing patients' comorbidities as necessary, in particular to optimize each patient's medical status before surgical procedures are performed.

The pretreatment evaluation at the Cleveland Clinic is consistent with published guidelines [7]. Because obese individuals are at higher risk for cardiovascular disease, a baseline electrocardiogram is performed. Cardiology evaluation is obtained when there is evidence of heart disease based on clinical symptoms or EKG findings. A chest X-ray and baseline laboratory testing are performed, including a complete blood count, chemistry panel, liver function tests, thyroid function tests, and a lipid profile.

Obstructive sleep apnea frequently goes unrecognized in this patient population until a thorough history prompts further evaluation. Patients with symptoms of loud snoring, daytime hypersomnolence, or a neck circumference greater than 17 in. undergo polysomnography and, if positive, they are treated with nasal continuous positive airway pressure. Asthma and obesity hypoventilation syndrome are other severe pulmonary complications of obesity that require evaluation by a pulmonologist.

The high incidence of diabetes in our patients is addressed by endocrinology participating in our bariatric clinics. Dietary counseling and psychological testing are also required for patients being referred for bariatric surgery.

Lifestyle Modifications

According to the clinical guidelines published by the American College of Physicians, all patients with a BMI of 30 kg/m^2 or greater should be counseled intensively on lifestyle and behavioral modifications such as appropriate diet and exercise [8, 9]. An algorithm from the ACP for medically managing obesity is shown in Fig. 20.1 [8]. The patient's goals for weight loss should be individually determined and may encompass other related parameters, such as decreasing blood pressure or fasting blood glucose levels. When establishing realistic weight loss goals, it is important to realize that modest weight loss of 10–15% from baseline is sufficient to produce health benefits [10, 11].

General diet guidelines for achieving and maintaining a healthy weight include eating balanced, nutritious foods to avoid vitamin deficiencies. Avoiding foods that are high in fat and simple sugars should be emphasized. In addition, the American Dietetics Association and American Diabetes Association recommend educating patients regarding portion sizes and caloric content of foods. Referral to a registered dietician helps patients initiate and adhere to these dietary guidelines.

The protein sparing modified fast (PSMF), a very low carbohydrate diet, is also an option for patients who are not surgical candidates, who prefer nonsurgical weight management even if morbidly obese, or for presurgical patients who have a BMI greater than 55. A typical patient on this diet consumes less than 50 g of carbohydrates per day and approximately 1,200 kcal. This type of ketogenic diet has been shown to accelerate fat loss, preserve lean tissue, and favorably impact metabolic responses [12]. In rare instances, presurgical patients have lost sufficient weight to change their pathway from a surgical to nonsurgical option.

Every obese patient should develop an exercise regimen as a part of a comprehensive lifestyle modification plan. Although exercise alone does not induce great amounts of weight loss, moderate exercise decreases blood pressure, increases HDL, and reduces triglycerides. It also predicts maintaining weight loss and delaying the onset of type 2 diabetes [13]. The American College of Sports Medicine and the American Heart Association recommend 30 min of moderate exercise 5 days a week for cardiovascular health, up to 60 min/day most days of the week for maintenance of weight, and 90 min/day for achieving weight loss.

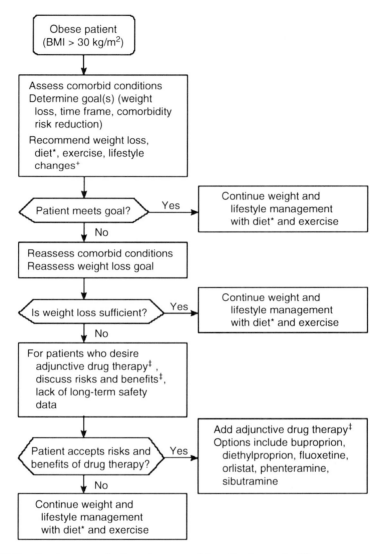

BMI = body mass index. Assess side effects and efficacy;
no data are available past 12 months except for orlistat.
Ann Int Med 2005;142 with permission

Fig. 20.1 Algorithm for the medical management of obesity

Medical Options

Pharmacologic therapy can be offered to obese patients who fail to achieve their weight loss goals through lifestyle modification alone, or have significant comorbidities. Before initiating therapy, patients must understand the drug's side effects, the lack of long-term safety data, and the temporary nature of the weight loss achieved with medications. Commonly used drugs include Sibutramine, Phentermine, Diethylpropion, and Orlistat. Orlistat was approved by the FDA in 2007 as an over-the-counter medication under the new name Alli, at half the strength of the original dose, 60 mg three times daily [14]. Then in October 2010, Abbott Laboratories, the manufacturer of Sibutramine, removed their drug from the U.S. market after FDA regulators stated it was too dangerous to use. This decision was based on results of a European study of cardiovascular outcomes in overweight and obese subjects, which showed an increased risk of heart disease and strokes in certain groups of treated patients [15]. Other drugs used for weight loss which are not FDA approved include Buproprion, Fluoxetine, Topiramate, and Zonisamide [8].

The choice of agent will depend on its side-effect profile and the patient's tolerance of these side effects. The amount of extra weight loss attributable to these medications is modest, <5 kg at 1 year. However, even modest weight loss, as seen with medical management, can slow the progression of diabetes and positively influence cardiovascular risk factors. There is no evidence, however, that modest weight loss affects mortality. The optimal duration of treatment with obesity medication has not been determined. Randomized, controlled trials have examined only 12 months of therapy, and there are no long-term data on whether these drugs decrease morbidity or mortality from obesity-related conditions. Thus, more long-term clinical trials are needed to answer these questions.

In selected patients who have had the laparoscopic adjustable gastric band (LAGB) procedure and have not lost 55% of their excess weight, a trial of a weight loss medicine is helpful. As an example, a 22-year-old patient who had the LAGB procedure was having difficulty reaching her target weight goal despite adherence to positive lifestyle and behavioral changes. After 6 months with minimal weight loss, and in spite of nearly reaching her band capacity for adjustments, she was placed on a 3-month trial of Phentermine. Her weight loss increased from 18 to 66 lbs during that time period. She reported significant enhancement of the LAGB effect in conjunction with the anoretic medicine, which motivated her to adhere more strongly to positive lifestyle changes and behaviors, even after she completed the medication trial.

Surgical Options

Indications. Patients with a BMI ≥35 kg/m² with obesity-related comorbidities and those with a BMI ≥40 kg/m² with or without comorbidities are eligible for bariatric surgery [1]. Patients must have attempted medical weight loss programs and should

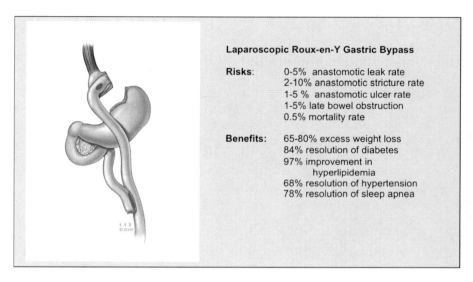

Laparoscopic Roux-en-Y Gastric Bypass

Risks: 0-5% anastomotic leak rate
               2-10% anastomotic stricture rate
               1-5 % anastomotic ulcer rate
               1-5% late bowel obstruction
               0.5% mortality rate

Benefits: 65-80% excess weight loss
               84% resolution of diabetes
               97% improvement in
                    hyperlipidemia
               68% resolution of hypertension
               78% resolution of sleep apnea

Fig. 20.2 Risks and benefits of Roux-en-Y gastric bypass

be highly motivated to change their lifestyle after surgery. The 1991 NIH guidelines recommended age limits between 18 and 60. At that time, there was insufficient evidence about surgery for patients outside of these limits. While advanced age is a predictor of increased mortality after bariatric surgery [16, 17], there is some evidence from case series to support bariatric surgery in carefully selected adolescents and elderly patients.

Contraindications. Patients who cannot tolerate general anesthesia due to cardiac, pulmonary, or liver diseases are not candidates for surgery. Additionally, patients must be able to understand the consequences of the surgery and comply with the extensive preoperative evaluation and the postoperative program that includes lifestyle changes, diet, vitamin supplementation, and medical follow-up. Patients who have ongoing substance abuse or unstable psychiatric illness are poor candidates for bariatric surgery.

Roux-en-Y Gastric Bypass. RYGB combines a restrictive and a malabsorptive procedure, and is the most common bariatric procedure performed in the United States (80%). Restrictive procedures reduce the stomach size, and malabsorptive procedures reduce the intestinal absorption of nutrients. The majority of RYGB cases are now performed laparoscopically, which results in faster recovery and fewer pulmonary and wound complications than open surgery. A small 15–30 cc gastric pouch is created to restrict food intake, and a Roux-en-Y anastomosis bypasses the duodenum and proximal jejunum, providing a malabsorptive component. The risks and benefits associated with RYGB are shown in Fig. 20.2. RYGB produces superior results compared to restrictive procedures with long-term excess weight reduction averaging 50% at 14 years, and improvements in comorbidities.

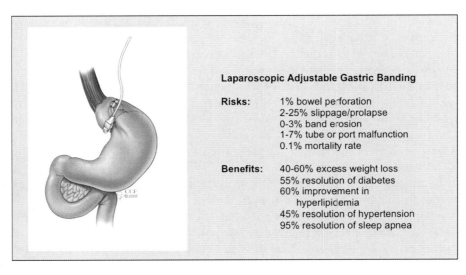

Laparoscopic Adjustable Gastric Banding

Risks: 1% bowel perforation
                 2-25% slippage/prolapse
                 0-3% band erosion
                 1-7% tube or port malfunction
                 0.1% mortality rate

Benefits: 40-60% excess weight loss
                 55% resolution of diabetes
                 60% improvement in
                    hyperlipidemia
                 45% resolution of hypertension
                 95% resolution of sleep apnea

Fig. 20.3 Risks and benefits of laparoscopic adjustable gastric band

Laparoscopic Adjustable Gastric Banding. The LAGB is a restrictive procedure. The device (Lap Band System, Inamed Health, Santa Barbara, California) was approved for use in the United States in 2001 after excellent results had been achieved in Europe and Australia. This silicone band with an inflatable inner collar is placed around the upper portion of the stomach to create a smaller gastric pouch. The band is connected to a subcutaneous port placed in the abdominal wall. Injecting or removing saline from the port adjusts the inner diameter of the band. Severe complications and mortality rates are lower for LAGB than RYGB, but LAGB typically results in less, and more gradual weight loss. Common risks and benefits of LAGB are shown in Fig. 20.3.

Biliopancreatic Diversion. BPD is a malabsorptive procedure performed by less than 3% of bariatric surgeons in the United States, but it is an option for a select number of supermorbidly obese patients (BMI greater than 100 kg/m^2) at the Cleveland Clinic. This procedure and a modification called the duodenal switch are designed to severely limit intestinal energy absorption. While this procedure offers the best and most durable weight loss of any bariatric procedure performed today, higher complication rates, nutritional deficiencies, and a higher mortality rate have limited its widespread use.

Laparoscopic Gastric Plication. A new innovation in 2011, LGP is still investigational as a primary procedure for weight loss. It is a restrictive procedure that involves sewing one or more large folds in the stomach wall to reduce the stomach volume. There is no cutting, stapling, or removal of the stomach or intestines during this procedure. It can also be reversed or converted to another procedure if needed. Patients are expected to lose 40–70% of their excess body weight in the first year after surgery. Risks are those common to any laparoscopic procedure, and major complications occur in less than 1% of patients.

Follow-up. Bariatric surgery patients require lifetime follow-up. Early postoperative visits focus on complications and the dramatic changes in dietary habits that result from restriction of stomach size. Later follow-up visits focus on medical and psychological support, nutritional assessment and vitamin supplementation, and adherence to exercise programs. Patients who present with new onset abdominal pain, vomiting, or gastroesophageal reflux months to years after bariatric surgery require reevaluation by their bariatric surgeon. These symptoms may be secondary to an anastomotic ulcer or stricture, or an intermittent bowel obstruction after RYGB. After LAGB, the new onset of gastroesophageal reflux or dysphagia may suggest gastric prolapse through the band.

In our practice, RYGB and BPD postoperative patients are seen the first week and first month by the surgeon, then every 3 months for the first year by our bariatrician with supportive visits to the dietician and psychologist when needed. The visit intervals then extend to 12–18 months. Diagnostic blood work is initially performed twice a year, and then once a year. Likewise, LAGB patients are seen within the first week and month, then every 6–12 weeks for ongoing band adjustments. All patients are encouraged to attend monthly support meetings.

Treatment Outcomes

Medical weight management outcomes in our bariatric practice are currently under review, and will be available in our 2011 outcomes book. The clinical trials results of anorectic medicines are published. Prior to being withdrawn from the market, a meta-analysis of Sibutramine in patients with a BMI of 25 kg/m^2 or greater showed that it was more effective than placebo in promoting weight loss in overweight and obese adults, with an average increased weight loss of 4.5 kg at 1 year compared to placebo [18, 19]. In a meta-analysis of 29 studies of Orlistat, the pooled mean weight loss for treated patients was 2.59 kg at 6 months and 2.89 kg at 12 months. The average age of patients enrolled was 48 years, and the average baseline BMI was 36.7 kg/m^2 [20].

Other agents such as Phentermine, Diethylpropion, and Fluoxetine result in 3.0–3.6 kg weight loss after 1 year when used in combination with lifestyle interventions. There is a paucity of data regarding Sertraline, Bupropion, Topiramate, and Zonsamide. Therefore, recommendations cannot be made until further studies are completed [21].

Our 2009 outcomes data shows that more than 65% of patients referred for bariatric surgery were either at high risk – body mass index greater than 50, or age 60 and over, or were referred for revisional bariatric procedures. The average preoperative body mass index for all patients in our surgical program in 2009 was 47.26 kg/m^2. More than 98% of our bariatric surgeries are performed laparoscopically. Despite their relatively high risk, less than 2% of our patients undergoing the two most common operations – laparoscopic gastric bypass and adjustable gastric banding – required postoperative ICU stays. The mean length of stay for both Roux-en-Y gastric bypass and adjustable gastric band procedures did increase in 2009 due to an increased number of high-risk patients.

In 2009, 60% of patients who had at least 18 months follow-up after bariatric surgery achieved more than 50% loss of their excess body weight, based on a normal body mass index of 25 kg/m². Twenty patients with type 2 diabetes mellitus underwent bariatric surgery in 2007, and had follow-up visits in 2008 and 2009. Their mean baseline hemoglobin A1c (HbA1c) was 8.1% (range 5.5–14.2) and mean baseline weight was 262 lbs (range 180–364). All but one patient took oral hypoglycemic medications before surgery with a range of two to four medications. Seven patients were also on insulin. On last follow-up, the mean weight loss in this cohort was 66 lbs (range 9–163), two patients remained on oral medications alone, and two remained on oral medications and insulin.

Our operative mortality for restrictive procedures, gastric bypass, and revision are 1.5%, 0.3%, and 0.0%, respectively. Mortality after bariatric surgery is primarily due to pulmonary embolism and anastomotic leaking. Complications of gastric bypass were relatively low, considering that more than 65% of these patients were at high risk from their disease and comorbidities. For 2008 and 2009, overall complications, anastomotic leak/stricture, and deep vein thrombosis/pulmonary embolus were less common than benchmarks for bariatric surgery [22].

Summary

As health care providers, we should be diligent in preventing and treating excess weight and obesity in our patients, and especially in preventing escalation of weight, as seen with patient William. We must educate patients regarding the medical consequences of their obesity, recognize that its origins are complex, then provide effective treatments, and monitor their progress. All overweight and obese patients should be counseled on lifestyle and behavioral modifications, such as appropriate diet and exercise. Pharmacologic therapy can be offered to those who have failed to lose weight with diet and exercise alone. When patients fail to lose excess weight, they should be offered referral to interdisciplinary weight loss programs. Bariatric surgery should be considered for morbidly obese patients who have failed medical weight loss programs – diet and exercise, with or without pharmacotherapy. Patients with a BMI higher than 40 kg/m², or higher than 35 kg/m² with obesity-related comorbidities, are candidates for bariatric surgery.

Editors' Comments: The Cleveland Clinic has integrated chronic disease management from traditional departmental approaches to interdisciplinary, system-based product lines across many diseases, and disease bundles. In this example of their obesity program, medical, surgical, and postsurgical management have been consolidated, and they are now moving into earlier prevention. Weight management is also a priority in their employee health program, and food services offer only healthy dietary options – no caloric sodas and no deep-fried foods. Their self-funded health plan realizes large dividends from addressing this important risk factor for hypertension, diabetes, heart disease, and kidney failure. JTH

References

1. NIH conference. Gastrointestinal surgery for severe obesity. Consensus Development Conference Panel. Ann Intern Med. 1991;115(12):956–61.
2. Ogden CL, Carroll MD, Curtin LR, et al. Prevalence of overweight and obesity in the United States, 1999–2004. JAMA. 2006;295(13):1549–55.
3. Wolf AM, Colditz GA. The cost of obesity: the US perspective. Pharmacoeconomics. 1994;5 Suppl 1:34–7.
4. Flegal KM, Graubard BI, Williamson DF, Gail MH. Excess deaths associated with underweight, overweight, and obesity. JAMA. 2005;293(15):1861–7.
5. Fontaine KR, Redden DT, Wang C, et al. Years of life lost due to obesity. JAMA. 2003; 289(2):187–93.
6. Third Report of the National Cholesterol Education Program (NCEP) Expert Panel on Detection, Evaluation, and Treatment of High Blood Cholesterol in Adults (Adult Treatment Panel III) final report. Circulation. 2002;106(25):3143–421.
7. Sauerland S, Angrisani L, Belachew M, et al. Obesity surgery: evidence-based guidelines of the European Association for Endoscopic Surgery (EAES). Surg Endosc. 2005;19(2):200–21.
8. Snow V, Barry P, Fitterman N, et al. Pharmacologic and surgical management of obesity in primary care: a clinical practice guideline from the American College of Physicians. Ann Intern Med. 2005;142(7):525–31.
9. McTigue KM, Harris R, Hemphill B, et al. Screening and interventions for obesity in adults: summary of the evidence for the U.S. Preventive Services Task Force. Ann Intern Med. 2003;139(11):933–49.
10. Pi-Sunyer FX. A review of long-term studies evaluating the efficacy of weight loss in ameliorating disorders associated with obesity. Clin Ther. 1996;18(6):1006–35. discussion 1005.
11. Harris MI, Flegal KM, Cowie CC, et al. Prevalence of diabetes, impaired fasting glucose, and impaired glucose tolerance in U.S. adults. The Third National Health and Nutrition Examination Survey, 1988–1994. Diabetes Care. 1998;21(4):518–24.
12. Volek JS, Westman EC. Very-low-carbohydrate weight-loss diets revisited. Cleveland Clinic J Med. 2002;69(11):849–62.
13. Knowler WC, Barrett-Connor E, Fowler SE, et al. Reduction in the incidence of type 2 diabetes with lifestyle intervention or metformin. N Engl J Med. 2002;346(6):393–403.
14. Rao G. Office-based strategies for the management of obesity. Am Fam Physician. 2010;81(12): 1429–49.
15. James WPT, Caterson ID, et al. Effect of Sibutramine on cardiovascular outcomes in overweight and obese subjects. N Engl J Med. 2010;363(10):905–17.
16. Flum DR, Salem L, Elrod JA, et al. Early mortality among Medicare beneficiaries undergoing bariatric surgical procedures. JAMA. 2005;294(15):1903–8.
17. Livingston EH, Huerta S, Arthur D, et al. Male gender is a predictor of morbidity and age a predictor of mortality for patients undergoing gastric bypass surgery. Ann Surg. 2002;236(5): 576–82.
18. Arterburn DE, Crane PK, Veenstra DL. The efficacy and safety of sibutramine for weight loss: a systematic review. Arch Intern Med. 2004;164(9):994–1003.
19. Haddock CK, Poston WS, Dill PL, et al. Pharmacotherapy for obesity: a quantitative analysis of four decades of published randomized clinical trials. Int J Obes Relat Metab Disord. 2002;26(2):262–73.
20. Sjostrom L, Lindroos AK, Peltonen M, et al. Lifestyle, diabetes, and cardiovascular risk factors 10 years after bariatric surgery. N Engl J Med. 2004;351(26):2683–93.
21. Wadden TA, Bartlett SJ, Foster GD, et al. Sertraline and relapse prevention training following treatment by very-low-calorie diet: a controlled clinical trial. Obes Res. 1995;3(6):549–57.
22. Nasr C, Rastgoufard S, Gamino R. Endocrinology and Metabolism Institute Outcomes 2009. Cleveland Clinic Foundation, 2010.

Chapter 21
Palliative Care and Hospice: Advancing the Science of Comfort, Affirming the Art of Caring

Martha L. Twaddle

Keywords Palliative care • Hospice • Biopsychosocial model • Hospice and palliative medicine • Science of comfort • End of life • Quality of life

Our greatest teachers are our patients – the professors whose robes open in the back. If we would just listen to their teachings, the wisdom born of experience, pain, weakness, and tenacity, we would hear what in healthcare really matters. The business of healthcare grows and has eclipsed the profession of providing care for the purpose of health and wellness. The physician/patient encounter, once sacred and full of the potential for healing has been distilled into a transaction. How long to treat the pneumonia, how many days should it take for you to be better? Why, the insurance company says just three. What are the outcomes that reflect quality? Less cost perhaps, and less time in the hospital. If I have delivered the cure by following this pathway, this protocol, why is it that you are not well? Why do you still tell me that you suffer when I prescribe the evidence-based medications, remove the tumors, dialyze the blood, staunch the bleeding? Why are you not well again? For wellness is not the outcome, but the journey. And the journey is one of companioning the ill all along the road, the journey is about the healer and the one who is ill, and how they teach one another.

The forced twilight of the shuttered room was heavy with the weariness of the unwashed and sleep deprived. Through the propped door the spirit of sadness abutted the din and glare of the nursing station. The interface as stark as a knife-edge, one side frenetically alive with white coats, rapid conversation, keyboards snapping as labs and medications are ordered, tests are reviewed, cases are discussed. The other dim lit territory holds the place of waiting, the absence of activity beyond labored

M.L. Twaddle, MD (✉)
Midwest Palliative and Hospice Care Center, Glenview, IL, USA
e-mail: mtwaddle@carecenter.org

J.T. Harrington and E.D. Newman (eds.), *Great Health Care: Making It Happen*, 199
DOI 10.1007/978-1-4614-1198-7_21, © Springer Science+Business Media, LLC 2012

breath and grunt-filled repositions, the antechamber to loss. Here in this room, the disease will not be vanquished. No procedures, treatments, or medications will change this outcome. Those suffused in the fluorescence of the nursing station are empty handed in offerings for this room, this patient, this family. They don't know what to do; they believe there is nothing to do. And so they ask me to come.

The shadowed forms of family members detach from the bedside, unfold and move slowly. Tissues clasped in hands, muffled coughs and throaty tears respond to my arrival. The spouse is an elderly man or perhaps just appears so; he is crumbled and compressed in the chair by the bedside, deflated with the anticipation of loss and the presence of grief. The patient, their loved one, lies already in state, sheets carefully folded across her skeletal chest which heaves and pauses in the labor of transition. Soft moans punctuate the rattle of secretions that pool in her throat, lips chapped and mouth dry, her head extended as though gulping air from a place of submersion.

I am asked to be here to speak of goals of care, symptom management, and decision-making regarding supportive options. But there is no time for the full exploration of palliative support. I will instead be the midwife for the death that is rapidly approaching.

I listen to their understanding and reflections; I hear their perceptions and their fears. I speak to them of the signs of comfort, and how we will ease this process for this woman they love. How tiny amounts of morphine in the cheek even now will smooth the brow and allow the shoulders to relax. How mouth care, done with her favorite soda, will moisten and remove the detritus upon her tongue; the family smiles with the idea, as perhaps there will be pleasure in this activity for both? Twin motion sickness patches behind the ears dry the rattle; music that she loved accompanies and softens the agonal vibrato. I explain the changes that will come, the mottling first on the knees, then spreading. How her face is the window of her experience – her smooth forehead and relaxed jaw reflects she does not suffer with the pauses and laboring of breath. I provide a timeframe for the travail – likely within the next many hours as her urination has ceased and her radial pulse is no longer present, her eyes cannot close completely and the rattle has begun. "It won't be long now. Are there any rituals and traditions that are important to you as a family to which we should be attentive? A chaplain, a priest, a rabbi, the iman, a spiritual guide, the friend, neighbor, sister; who should be called?"

Within this discussion, the family ignites again the spark of purpose, the sense of direction, the clarity of roles, and how they are helping the woman they love. Even her husband straightens perceptively in his chair – leans forward to whisper in her ear and lay his head by hers on the pillow, knowing this helps, knowing there is something to do. Paperwork for hospice may seem intrusive – yet this provides the door to more support, more for this family beyond the death. "The grandchildren will need bereavement support, the visit from the hospice nurse will be so helpful for our mother...oh yes, could the chaplain come? You have a music therapist?" Tears flow afresh but they are different now, a relief expressed, so much that can be done, so much that can help – what a bountiful outpouring of support and companionship. "Thank you so much for coming. Thank you thank you..." And that last sentence said time and again, "Why didn't we know about you sooner?"

Martha L. Twaddle

Why Do We Wait?

These scenarios of late hospice referrals were my steady diet in the early years of this work and sadly, they even occur today. The median length of stay for patients utilizing the Medicare Hospice Benefit is still hovering around 21 days [1]. Physicians not understanding the full purpose of hospice, coupled with the tendency to wait until the prognosis is clearly end-stage, delay assessments for hospice such that they are "brink of death" referrals [2, 3]. In the 22 years that I have done this work, families have repeated the mantra of "why didn't we have this sooner; where were you 6 months ago?" even as the physicians say, "They aren't ready for hospice yet!"

Very early in this work, I asked myself the same – why do we wait? Why do we wait for death to be imminent to discuss quality of life and the needs of the patient and family beyond just the treatment of the disease? Treating the disease is often described as a battle, but why is it that we risk collateral damage to the patient and family in an all-out press to annihilate the illness? I recognized early the current culture of medicine is one of exhaustion – exhausting interventional options, treatments, finances, and the people and then, after the last attempt is made and all are truly spent, saying, *"we have nothing left to offer you."* This is the warrior mentality – the effort and the struggle until the defeat – whether death or the mortification of surrender.

In truth there is always something that can be done. Much can be done to support the patient and family weathering the illness, even when cure is a phantasmal goal. Although there may be no more disease-specific interventions, there is always much to do. Perhaps the treatment of the disease directly is too toxic or burdensome, yet the referral of the patient to palliative care and support would add quality and even quantity to life. Most often there are symptoms: physical, psychological, and spiritual manifestations of the distress of living with serious and life-threatening illness. The easing of the symptoms themselves, the palliation, can translate into improvements in well-being evidenced by enhanced function, appetite, cognition, and perceived well-being. Anecdotally and now evidenced by peer-reviewed articles, patients who received interdisciplinary palliative support live longer and with better quality than those who receive only disease-focused medical care [4, 5]. In essence, patients and families do better when receiving care based on a biopsychosocial model than a biomedical model alone. This is by no means a new discovery. In truth, it resonates with Plato's initial philosophy of allopathic medicine.

The support of hospice is more than the warm companionship of kind people. It has grown into a profession with demonstrated benefits in enhancing quality of life. From the standpoint of patients and their families, hospice care has better outcomes in the control of symptoms such as pain than routine medical care, and high patient/family satisfaction is consistently reported [6, 7]. From the standpoint of the bereaved, evidence now demonstrates that the surviving spouse is less likely to become ill or die if they received hospice care [8]. Bereavement support, typically provided for over a year after the death, significantly reduces the risk of complicated grief [9]. In essence, hospice serves the public health – a good death is preventative medicine for the bereaved.

But why do we wait to practice the biopsychosocial model? Why is this approach reserved for those in the end stages of disease, whether malignant or chronic? There is no benefit to waiting to access supportive care, and mounting evidence to suggest that so much could be done that will provide benefit, even while a serious illness is being treated or a progressive chronic condition is being managed. In my formative years in the practice of medicine, I felt passionately that there must be a way to wed the benefits of hospice care (the biopsychosocial spiritual model) with the treatment of the disease, such that these modalities might occur simultaneously in the care of the seriously ill, and literally complement one another. I sensed, however, that the idea of extending the support of hospice upstream from the end of life could not be uniquely mine.

My first intersection was at a gathering of the International Hospice Institute and Academy of Hospice Physicians in Estes Park Colorado in 1990. The IHI/AHP was created by Drs. Josephina Magno and Gerald Holman in 1988 as a means to bring together the thought leaders in this field, as well as to facilitate the emerging professional identity of those committed to this critical area of health care [10]. What affirmation for me to recognize the like-minded professionals who identified hospice care as their vocation and within that tribe, Dr. Balfour Mount from McGill University. As a urologic surgeon from McGill who had then further studied at Memorial Sloan Kettering for surgical oncology, and trained additionally with Dame Cicely Saunders, the founder of the hospice movement, Bal was demonstrating in his work that the idea of the interdisciplinary model of hospice care could be applied from the time of diagnosis throughout the trajectory of a serious illness. He called this approach Palliative Care, and its professional discipline, Palliative Medicine.

Palliative Care at Northwestern

The initial efforts to emulate Bal's model in the American healthcare system were at Northwestern Memorial Hospital (NMH) in Chicago, the farsighted design of Drs. Charles von Gunten and Jamie von Roenn. All who had the privilege to work with them considered the addition of a "von" to their own name. In the early "1990s," Drs. Von Gunten and von Roenn created a Palliative Care Unit and consult service to provide assistance to seriously ill patients and their families throughout the larger hospital complex. The Palliative Care Unit resided in the fading grandeur of Passavant Hospital, one of the original institutions that joined with Wesley Hospital to form NMH in the early 1970s. Passavant's dark wood-paneled foyers and soaring

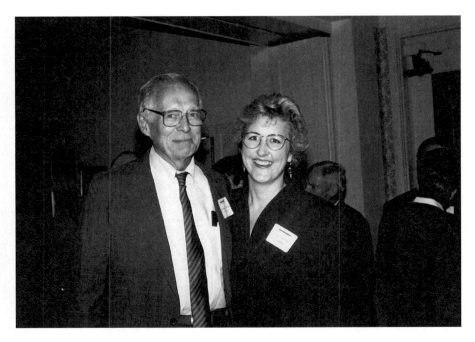

Fig. 21.1 Dr. Martha Twaddle with her mentor Dr. Harry Miller, Northwestern University Feinberg School of Medicine in the 1990s

ceilings with their crown moldings and medallions lent an air of dignity and fading refinement to the care of the very ill, and those who were dying. The initiation of the service coincided with the years of the AIDs epidemic, and many of the patients receiving care in the Palliative Care Unit suffered the ravages of this disease. However, Palliative Care extended its benefit far beyond the structured unit setting to serve patients throughout the hospital – on the oncology ward, the cardiology, renal, and intensive care units, and in the emergency room. The benefit of the Palliative Care team's expertise in symptom control and their effective communication skills in negotiating complex medical decision-making became widely known and utilized for patients and families regardless of diagnosis or prognosis. Within the academic programming of NMH, the Palliative Care Service became a sought after teaching rotation, especially for those physicians-in-training who were pursuing a career in oncology (Fig. 21.1).

The success of the Palliative Care Service model at NMH served as the archetype for a service at the Evanston Hospital, Northwestern's then North Side cousin, in 1995. With the business leadership of Dorothy Pitner, the CEO and President of the Hospice of the North Shore, I initiated a Palliative Care Consultation Service in Evanston Hospital in 1994, followed by the creation of a specialty hospice unit in 1995, and an associated educational program. Like the flagship downtown, this service grew rapidly and integrated into the day-to-day functions of the teaching hospital.

The Palliative Care Service was asked to see patients facing the end of life and needing hospice services, but increasingly was sought to help with the complex care needs of the chronically ill – those experiencing increasing disease-related infirmities and actively engaged in the treatment of their disease – with the hope of improved function, remission, or cure.

Most frequently, the role of Palliative Care was to facilitate the patient's and family's understanding of the illness and its natural history and prognosis, clarify how the patient and family defined quality of life, and assist in complex medical decision-making informed by the context of patient and family values. These time-intensive discussions were, and are, the day-to-day activity of the Palliative Care interdisciplinary team. The growth and success of these early models within the greater Northwestern system were mirrored across the nation. By 2006, more than 50% of hospitals larger than 50 beds reported a palliative care program [11].

"Martha, what can I tell you?" Her voice held the richness of coffee, the nuances of dark chocolate. Sultry, smooth, her Columbian accent caressed her spoken English as she related to me the current updates of proposed treatments and findings. Sophie had been my teacher in my early years of residency, an intimidating and fast paced preceptor in the University Student Health Clinic. She suffered no slackers and was intolerant of any resident who intimated that this rotation might be a time to relax after the grueling months of inpatient care. In those weeks of ambulatory care, I don't recall her smiling, except with patients. Rather, there was the scrutiny, the side-glance squinted gaze with a slight uplift of the eyebrows that monitored my interactions and assessments. Did I measure up?

Imagine the leap of my viscera when after my first few years in the practice of primary care internal medicine, Sophie's name appeared on my new patient list. The shift from trainee to physician, from student to teacher and guide, is a role change that evoked a sense of awe and gratitude, a profoundly powerful communication of trust and mutual respect. No patient is ever taken for granted, and especially those who have taught us the art and craft of medicine. The emphasis on the sacred relationship, and trust, the core of healing in medicine, is captured in this moment of selection.

Within years, Sophie's and my journey was punctuated by my diagnosing her breast cancer by mammography and palpation. Lumpectomy and sentinel node biopsy revealed that she had Stage IIB breast cancer and would require both radiation and chemotherapy. She struggled with the treatment, suffering significant drops in her white count without the expected rebound, and often requiring hospitalization for neutropenic fever. Sophia's completion of treatment and recovery coincided with my decision to devote my entire medical career to Palliative Medicine, leaving primary care internal medicine for this specialty practice. I recall Sophie's proclamation that "I will come with you; I am a Palliative Care patient."

She established care with a topnotch internist in the area, another of her prior students, and came to see me soon after the transition regarding pain in her knee. Given her very recent journey with breast cancer, we feared the worst and were even more leveled by the discovery that the new lesion in her distal femur, and explanation for her persistent low white blood cell count, was multiple myeloma. What followed were 4 years of a progressive, chronic illness with the intense symptom burden of treatments and the disease itself.

But what eclipsed the disease in those 4 years of illness was a life lived fully: international travel, social activity, rich enjoyment of family, friends, and community. Sophie's oncologist commented to me "I think she has lived so well and so long because of Palliative Care." Sophie's illness culminated in her admission to inpatient hospice care, just as she had requested and planned years prior to the day. She died comfortably with her family and friends at her side – no unnecessary crisis, no damaging drama, but rather a comfortable and respectful ending of the life of a much-loved woman.

Fitting that Sophie, instrumental in my ambulatory medicine education, would be the trailblazer of my Palliative Medicine specialty practice. Throughout the 1990s and in the early years of twenty-first century, Palliative Care was primarily a hospital-based consultation service. The Center for the Advancement of Palliative Care, brought into being by the creative genius of Dr. Diane Meier, was wildly successful in modeling and mentoring the creation of inpatient Palliative Care specialty services across the country [12]. Our initial emphasis at Midwest Care Center was also hospital-based, an upstream continuum with hospice care. As one of Diane's early faculty, I helped develop and teach about the synergy of community-based hospice programs partnering with hospitals in the creation of the specialty service of palliative medicine, and the interdisciplinary expression of this discipline called Palliative Care. Our Palliative Care consult service grew to serve five area hospitals and three distinct healthcare systems.

Why Palliative Care?

As the practice of medicine was becoming increasingly location based, our team of specialists would, in contrast, follow the seriously ill across the continuum from hospital to nursing home to home and back again as necessary. As my colleagues increasingly defined their scope of practice to include a setting of care – whether as hospitalists, nursing home physicians, or office-based clinicians – we were asked to maintain continuity of care for those with advanced chronic illness regardless of where they were. What followed over the years were referrals and consultation requests from other physicians to help with symptom management, to facilitate the complex decision-making about upcoming treatments, to reassess prognosis, and to provide understanding of the anticipated outcomes of the disease(s) to patients and families. These consultations were needed in all settings of care – the hospital, long-term care settings, in the home and office. What my colleagues needed from us and what we could provide were expertise in communication skills and continuity of care across sites of care and time.

As physicians' productivity requirements drove them to see more patients by limiting appointments to 15 min and lengthening their workdays, what they needed increasingly from Palliative Care was help – help in all settings of care with addressing and orchestrating care delivery for the complex needs of their patients and families struggling with the progression of serious chronic illness and debility. What patients and families wanted and needed from us, struggling as they did in our fragmented healthcare system, was regular time-intensive discussions to understand their illness and its consequences, and the continuity across sites of care delivery, so particularly when they were weakened and infirm, they had a professional advocate with whom they had established trust. Truly, what they needed from us, and continue to need, was the best of health care – healing relationships that endure across time and space.

Over the past 30 years, the rapid causes of death have declined, while gradual causes have grown exponentially. Most people today do not die suddenly, they die incrementally. The delivery of health care, from staffing to billing, is organized around institutions instead of patients. Gradual dying is treated as a medical crisis instead of a natural process.

Stephen Kiernan, *Last Rights; Rescuing The End of Life from the Medical System* 2006.

"We need to focus less on doing things to *you and more on doing things* for *you."* Jeff Zilberstein, MD, Intensivist, Northwest Community Hospital, meeting with a patient and family.

Patients with chronic illnesses and their families are ill-served by a system that focuses only on crisis-intervention and defines medical care only by an intervention or procedure and by the site of the encounter, but these are exactly the criteria that determine physicians' billings and revenues. As the economy of medicine has deteriorated such that primary care physicians can no longer afford to leave their offices, and as patients move from one primary physician to another as employment-related health plans dictate, the care of the chronically ill has become increasingly fragmented and subjected to overutilization. Now when Mrs. Smith, 89 years of age, is admitted again with her progressive dementia, obstructive lung disease, cor pulmonale, and heart failure, her internist or family medicine physician is ensconced in his or her office, often unaware that a crisis has even occurred. A cadre of specialists then sweep into action; Mrs. Smith, once a person, mother, grandmother, is disintegrated into her organ systems and a specialist is assigned to each. The anxious daughter at her bedside beseeches "how is my mother?" and each specialist reports on her or his expertise in restoring the function of their respective body part. Mrs. Smith is not just the sum total of her physical parts; the restoration of physical function does not confirm that Mrs. Smith is well, and the "medically indicated" procedures and protocols incited by her admission may become, as Eric Cassell said in 1982, *"the source of suffering itself"* [13].

Palliative Care seeks to reintegrate the person through expertise in the biopsychosocial approach of health care, and to better ascertain through attentive communication what constitutes a meaningful healthcare outcome. The results of this perspective, the comprehensive assessments and the discussions that follow, are that patients and families have a greater understanding of the burdens and benefits of treatments and procedures, and will more frequently focus or limit medical interventions to those that are most likely to improve their quality of life [14].

Barriers to Providing Palliative Care

How is it that we as Palliative Care consultants can spend the time in these discussions when other physician cannot? In part, it is the communication expertise that is finely honed in those who practice in this discipline. The abilities to "break the bad news" or to facilitate an emotionally charged family meeting are the critical competencies of any Palliative Care practitioner. In addition, Palliative Care is defined and practiced by interdisciplinary teams – physicians working in collaboration with advanced practice nurses, nurses, social workers, chaplains, and other professionals. The thorough discussions around advance care planning require time, thoughtful explanations, and skill. These are the day-to-day "procedures" for which we are trained, and we can provide them with focus, effectiveness, and efficiency. And the interdisciplinary approach allows greater expertise for all aspects of biopsychosocial care.

Sadly, our current healthcare remuneration does not support this care model. More reimbursement is provided for placing an arterial catheter than facilitating a 60-min family meeting. Attempts to legislate the funding of these critical patient and family care interventions have been thwarted by the gross misperception that this insurance benefit would support "death panels." If labeling is necessary, palliative care teams are "quality of life defenders."

We, as Palliative Care professionals, can typically only exist by being part of a greater entity, such as a nonprofit community-based program, or by relying, quite honestly, on the business of hospice care to support the business of palliative care. Although we can demonstrate efficient and effective utilization of limited resources, cost savings to patients/families and hospital systems, highly effective symptom management that often translates into earlier discharge from inpatient to outpatient settings, and high patient/family satisfaction, what we have yet to achieve is a sustainable model of palliative care as a stand-alone entity. The very issues that prevented our primary care colleagues from provisioning this time-intensive care, its associated cost and lack of reimbursement, are as real for us. We can financially partner our service with hospitals, long-term care facilities, and with hospice programs to create an economically sustainable model. Even so, the finances are a challenge, particularly for providing interdisciplinary Palliative Care outside of the hospital.

The Emergence of the American Academy of Hospice and Palliative Medicine

But the intention of Palliative Care was never to be just another medical specialty in a "stand alone" model. In the early 1990s at a breakfast meeting in Chicago, the intention was set to pursue specialty recognition for Palliative Medicine. The reason for this lofty pursuit was not only to secure recognition of the discipline's competencies and contributions to health care, but also to spur more research of interventions for care models for the seriously ill and at the end of life. It was first and foremost to infiltrate medical education – to insure that every practicing physician was again schooled in the biopsychosocial model of patient/family centered care. Curricula specific to communication skills and caring for the imminently dying patient would become requirements in medical school and residency programs. Medical students would be evaluated regarding the knowledge, skills, and behaviors in how to best care for patients and families with advanced chronic illness and at the end of life.

The official specialty of Hospice and Palliative Medicine (HPM) is supported by ten cosponsoring Boards, unprecedented in medical history. Whether a surgeon,

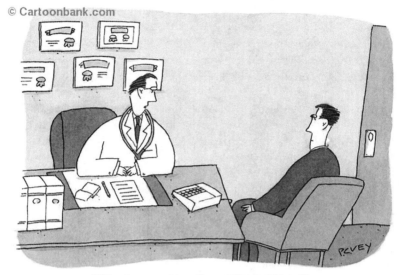

*"There's no easy way I can tell you this, so I'm
sending you to someone who can."*

Fig. 21.2 Courtesy of author MLT

neurologist, obstetrician, emergency room physician, pediatrician, physiatrist, family medicine physician, internist, psychiatrist, radiologist, or anesthesiologist, one can seek further specialty training in this field and likewise, the primary certification exams for each discipline now contain questions reflective of the HPM competencies (Fig. 21.2).

Now more than 4 years after specialty recognition, the profession of Hospice and Palliative Medicine seeks through mentoring, modeling, and formal education to further drive the development of primary and specialty levels of palliative care. Through the creation of evidence-based pathways, primary palliative interventions can be set into motion throughout a health system. A patient with aspiration pneumonia admitted to the hospital from a nursing home sparks an immediate review of advance directives and a family meeting with an interdisciplinary team to review how the patient/family unit defines meaningful care and outcomes. Taken one step further, patients living in nursing homes with advanced serious illness can be identified proactively for interdisciplinary assessment and family conferences around goals of care and complex medical decision-making. These early discussions allow patients and families to select and advocate for those care interventions that are most consistent with their definition of quality of life, and to avoid interventions that would not provide meaningful benefit or cause suffering.

All members of healthcare teams, regardless of the site of care, can be taught and mentored in effective communication techniques, primary symptom management skills, and cultural sensitivity. Palliative Care education can be, and in many ways, intends to be the means to resurrect the principles of holistic healthcare.

A Work in Progress and Progress from Our Work

As per the motto of the American Academy of Hospice and Palliative Medicine: "*Advancing the Science of Comfort, Affirming the Art of Caring*," this area of health care is vitally important to all of us, as healthcare providers and as patients ourselves. Over the past 10 years, the demographics of patients utilizing the Medicare Hospice Benefit have gradually and steadily changed. Once a benefit used predominantly by end-stage cancer patients, now more than 70% of hospice patients have such diagnoses as Dementia, Congestive Heart Failure, Chronic Obstructive Pulmonary Disease, Chronic Kidney Disease, etc. The other significant shift in utilization of the benefit has been the increasing length of stay in Hospice Care for patients with these diagnoses. As they have benefitted from the biopsychosocial model, they have thus lived with quality much longer than their initially anticipated limited prognosis. These patients and families then graduate out of Hospice, and yet they still very much require an active attentive case management-based healthcare program.

The transitions in and out of Hospice Care are inherently challenging, given the departure of the hospice nurse case-manager, and the required shifts in medication coverage and equipment. These upheavals can take a significant toll on patients and families, risking the unintended acute crisis if care delivery is not carefully coordinated. Here is another area of significant Palliative Care need and involvement; one of my patients went in and out of her Medicare Hospice Benefit three times over approximately 8-year period before her final readmission and death.

Conclusion

Again, those who teach us what is the best in health care are those who receive and judge our professional offerings: our patients and their families. We are in the business of taking care of people, and we must focus on that as well as the eradication of the disease. At some point, the disease will no longer be one we can "fix" and the attempts to do so will risk the waste of the patient's precious time and energy, of the health system's resources, and of everyone's money. In the final phases, it is about living well in spite of advanced chronic illness, it is about being "at ease" in spite of the disease, such that we can focus on the life we have and what matters most. Palliative Care and Hospice care are the means to make this possible.

Editor's Comments: Martha Twaddle provided so much that was entirely new to me, and from such a sensitive perspective. I felt like I was present at the birth of her specialty, and I admire the broad educational mission of Palliative Care specialists beyond training more of their own. Like our other champions, they have reached out to other providers to help patients together. Of the many provocative questions Martha raises, we need to take ownership of the disparity between value delivered by palliative care teams and current reimbursement, similar to what Dick Leuker and Beth McCormick described for cardiac rehabilitation. Investments in these high value and relatively inexpensive services would be recaptured easily by reducing more costly, ineffective care, and improving patients' and families quality of life and productivity. Insurance companies focused on annual profits just don't care. When will we learn? JTH

References

1. 2010 Edition of NHPCO facts and figures: Hospice care in America. http://www.nhpco.org/files/public/Statistics_Research/Hospice_Facts_Figures_Oct-2010.pdf. Accessed February 22, 2011.
2. Lamont EB, Christakis NA. Physician factors in the timing of cancer patient referral to hospice palliative care. Cancer. 2002;94:2733–7.
3. Kiernan SP. Rescuing the end-of-life from the medical system. New York: St. Martin's Press; 2006.
4. Christakis NA, Escarce JE. Survival of Medicare patients after enrollment in hospice programs. N Engl J Med. 1996;335:172–8.
5. Temel JS, Greer JA, Muzikansky A, et al. Early palliative care for patients with metastatic non-small-cell lung cancer. N Engl J Med. 2010;363:733–42.
6. Connor SR, Teno J, Spence C, Smith N. Family evaluation of hospice care: results from voluntary submission of data via website. J Pain Symptom Manage. 2005;30:9–17.
7. Connor SR, Tecca M, LundPerson J, Teno J. Measuring hospice care: The National Hospice and Palliative Care Organization National Hospice Data Set. J Pain Symptom Manage. 2004; 28:316–28.
8. Christakis NA, Iwashyna TJ. The health impact of healthcare on families: a matched cohort study of hospice use by decedents and mortality outcomes in surviving, widowed spouses. Soc Sci Med. 2003;57:465–75.
9. Lautrette A, Darmon M, Megarbane B, et al. A communication strategy and brochure for relatives of patients dying in the ICU. N Engl J Med. 2007;356:469–78.
10. History of the American Academy of Hospice and Palliative Medicine. http://www.aahpm.org/about/default/history.html. Accessed February 22, 2011.
11. Nelson R. Palliative care programs continue to increase in American hospitals. http://www.medscape.com/viewarticle/720534. Accessed February 22, 2011.
12. Center to Advance Palliative Care. http://www.capc.org/about-capc. Accessed April 3, 2011.
13. Cassel EJ. The nature of suffering and the goals of medicine. N Engl J Med. 1982;306:639–45.
14. Gade G, Venohr I, Conner D, et al. Impact of an inpatient palliative care team: a randomized control trial. J Palliat Med. 2008;11:180–90.

Part V
Controversies in Redesigning Chronic Disease Care

J. Timothy Harrington

What we've got here is ... failure to communicate (The Captain, in Cool Hand Luke, 1967).

False dilemma: Wikipedia – The logical fallacy of false dilemma also known as falsified dilemma, fallacy of the excluded middle, black and white thinking, false dichotomy, false correlative, either/or fallacy and bifurcation involves a situation in which two alternative points of view are held to be the only options, when in reality there exist one or more other options which have not been considered.

Listen! Learn to be an interested and attentive listener. Since almost all people are attracted to those who are interested in them – and good listeners are rare and in great demand – this is the most important social skill you can develop. It feels great to have someone interested in you. To be a good listener, maintain eye contact rather than looking around the room. Stay on him. Do not bring the subject back to you after he pauses. Rather, let him continue and encourage him to talk more by asking follow-up questions like "Why?" or "How come?" or "Tell me more." Avoid the social sin of interrupting so that you can say what you think or know (Dick Goldberg, Clinical Psychologist, in The 10 Simple Secrets to Being Liked by Almost Everybody, © 2006).

In this final part, let's explore several controversies that are barriers to creating great health care – to health care stakeholders coming together to solve problems. Too often we strive to prevail against others whose interests and beliefs we view as conflicting with our own instead of working together for patients' and the public's interests. Self-interest, unfounded beliefs, disregard for objective information,

J.T. Harrington, MD
Division of Rheumatology, University of Wisconsin School of Medicine and Public Health, Madison, WI, USA

polarization, and a "failure to communicate" dominate the health care dialogue, like so much of our broader National discourse. Finding solutions will require a different approach: examining the data and other objective information, defining problems rationally, and working together to solve them. We need to begin listening to each other if health care is to become what it needs to be. We can't afford to do otherwise.

Chapter 22
Myths and Miscreants

Eric D. Newman

Keywords Myths • Miscreants • Journey • Generalizable • Quality • Non-adoptors • Diffusion of innovations • Adoption • Innovators

Even us die-hard redesigners at times exhibit non-adopter behaviors. For me, it was dancing. The very word would throw me into an apoplectic fit. While I enjoyed music, I suffered from a cosmetically embarrassing case of 3 left feet. However, since I could count to "4," my wife Laurie felt I had sufficient knowledge to learn how to swing dance.

Well, wouldn't you know it, Bloomsburg University was conveniently offering a Swing Dance course, and Laurie wanted us to attend. Together, no less! I fought her tooth and nail – typical non-adopter behaviors. It's too early; it's too late; I am different (well, 1 out of 3 was correct). Laurie dragged me, kicking and screaming, to the first Swing Dance lesson. I quickly noted several things:

1. *I really could count to 4. In fact, apparently I counted to 4 out loud for the first 10 lessons.*
2. *I only had two left feet, and on rare occasion, just one.*
3. *My wife liked to lead. I liked to step on her toes, sometimes just for fun.*
4. *I actually started to enjoy myself.*

After several months of lessons, we both "graduated," and were awarded a Swing Dance Course Certificate from Bloom U – I had it mounted and hung on my exam room wall, next to my other medical education certificates. Patients apparently liked this – "Oh he's a well-trained doctor, AND he has rhythm."

We became serious about dancing. A group of us started a local chapter of USABDA (United States Amateur Ballroom Dancers Association). We held monthly dances, complete with lessons and a live band, for over 15 years. The guys bought tuxedos and colorful cummerbunds – the gals an assortment of sparkly gowns. We met many wonderful dancing friends, and could swing, rhumba, cha-cha, and tango with the best of them. We gained a lifetime of stories, experiences, and friendships (Fig. 22.1).

E.D. Newman, MD (✉)
Department of Rheumatology, Clinical Innovations, Division of Medicine,
Geisinger Health System, Danville, PA, USA
e-mail: arthman@aol.com

J.T. Harrington and E.D. Newman (eds.), *Great Health Care: Making It Happen*,   213
DOI 10.1007/978-1-4614-1198-7_22, © Springer Science+Business Media, LLC 2012

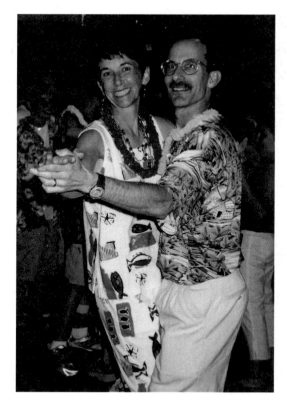

Fig. 22.1 "Let's Do the Lindy Hop"

> *If I had continued in my non-adopter behaviors, I would never have known what I could accomplish. To quote Wayne Gretsky – "You miss 100% of the shots you never take."*
> *Take a chance. Or two. The worst that happens is your wife leads.*
>
> *Eric D. Newman*

This chapter covers 2 forces that slow our progress to improve healthcare delivery: (1) misconceptions about quality improvement ("myths"), and (2) nonadopter behaviors performed by nonadopters ("miscreants," in its broadest sense of nonbelievers). Dispelling the myths to understand about how innovations actually spread through human systems is critical to improvement. Understanding nonadaptors who undermine innovation by their very nature is as well.

First Myths. There are many myths and misconceptions about what quality improvement work is and what it can accomplish. Here are but a few myths that are worth exploring.

Myth #1: Quality is a destination.
Truth #1: Quality is a journey.

Improving quality is a journey of enlightenment – learning, exploring, and making lives better in a continuous iterative (repetitive) fashion. Many institutions consider quality improvement as a specific project with a set goal. Once the goal is achieved, another project is taken on, and the original project is left to survive on its own. Since we know that systems are unruly and follow chaos theory, the end result is slippage of quality, work performed for no lasting purpose. Successful institutions will continue to readdress goals and spend time and effort continuing to measure the success or slippage of important projects. If it's important enough to improve, it's important enough to track and to sustain.

Myth #2: Quality improvement is not generalizable.
Truth #2: Quality improvement is in fact more generalizable than the knowledge gained by randomized controlled trials and effectiveness research.

Quality improvement is continuous learning and change in "real-world" environments. The work done locally can indeed be "scaled up." A striking example is the Fracture Liaison Service that begun in 1999 by Alastair McLellan as a local osteoporosis improvement program in West Glasgow, Scotland [1]. His team focused on patients who had already sustained a fragility fracture, an underserved population with a high risk of further fractures and a high price tag, not just in Glasgow, but everywhere. Over a decade, this highly successful program has processed 9,000 new fracture patients per year in Greater Glasgow alone and has expanded throughout Scotland, Wales, Ireland, and Great Britain. If expansion from a local program to an international, policy-changing adoption doesn't demonstrate quality improvement work being generalizable, I don't know what does! We will examine this myth again in Chap. 24.

Myth #3: Quality can be thought, bought, and taught.
Truth#3: Ehhhhh. Wrong, at least partially.

Quality can be thought refers to the misconception that quality is something that you "know," and hence does not need to be measured. "I know good quality, and I provide it," is simply unacceptable when dealing with human needs and using finite resources. You don't understand what you don't measure.

Quality can be bought refers to the age-old tactic of hiring outside contractors to do the job. An external quality SWAT team can indeed swoop in, reorganize people, places and processes, and improve quality of care. And when they leave, people are left angry, the processes fall apart, cats mate with dogs, and general brouhaha ensues. For improvement to be sustainable, the process needs to be *owned* by the participants, not thrust upon them by outsiders.

My identifying *Quality can be taught* as a myth may confuse you. After all, isn't that what this book is about? We can teach the methodology to you, your team, your institution, and your system, but quality improvement has to be lived. You have to get out there, get dirty, kick the tires, and take QI for a spin. Far too often we have seen individuals and groups attend redesign or quality improvement seminars and courses, only to return to their harried "stamp out today's fires" lives and never practice what they learned. They may not take the time and make the effort, or they may just be overwhelmed. That's precisely why we emphasize trying out the techniques on a small scale and trying, "failing," learning, and trying again. PDSA.

Previous chapters have focused on other myths and misconceptions about process redesign to improve quality, but the corresponding truths are worth recapitulating:

- Your view from your vantage is skewed and may be wrong. Don't judge in haste as you solve problem; seek a more robust view.
- You are not an island unto yourself. You work in a system. Your actions, or lack thereof, have significant upstream and downstream consequences.
- Your staff has better ideas than you do. Empower them to be heard, and listen to them.
- You don't understand what you don't measure – enough said.
- Complaining is easy – change is hard!

Now for miscreants. Miscreants, aka nonadoptors, account for a small percentage of society, but they stand out, and they seem to congregate in healthcare. Nonadopters obstruct any and all change, causing unending grief, aggravation, and gastritis for those trying to lead and participate in effecting it. They hold tightly to their myths and misunderstandings. They defend the status quo. They can do so passively by ignoring required tasks, or actively through their verbal and physical actions. The challenge for leadership and other is to put improvement ahead of keeping the peace with those who resist progress. For many organizations, this will require breaking traditions of mollifying these nonadapters among us.

Nonadopters, like birds, are easy to identify once you listen to their vocalizations, such as:

- We're too busy.
- It won't work.
- We don't have enough staff, space, paperclips, etc.
- We're special.
- Everyone else is doing it this way.
- We have been doing it this way for years.
- People wait to see me because I am that good.
- We have too many other commitments.
- Quality Improvement is the flavor of the month.
- This is just about administration trying to get me to see more patients.

And my favorite…

- You're just rearranging chairs on the Titanic.

To best understand the nonadopter in his/her native habitat, we need to discuss how new ideas spread and are adopted (or not). This area of study is known as diffusion of innovations. Everett M. Rogers, PhD, developed the conceptual foundation for this field. He was a sociologist whose work spanned 4 decades – from 1960 through the 1990s. His seminal book, Diffusion of Innovations, was first published in 1962 [2]. Dr. Rogers defined the elements required for diffusion of an innovation, the characteristics of the innovation, the process that occurs as an innovation is adopted (or not), and the adopter categories of those humans involved (Table 22.1).

Table 22.1 Diffusion of innovation key concepts

Elements	Innovation
	Communication channels
	Time
	Social system
Characteristics	Relative advantage
	Compatibility
	Complexity
	Trialability
	Observability
Process	Knowledge
	Persuasion
	Decision
	Implementation
	Confirmation
Adopter categories	Innovators
	Early adopters
	Early majority
	Late majority
	Laggards

According to Dr. Rogers' work, there are four key elements in the diffusion process:

1. *Innovation* – defined as a concept, entity, or process that is viewed as new by those who need to adopt it.
2. *Communication channels* – defined as the route used to communicate from one person to another.
3. *Time* – defined in terms of time to move through the innovation process, as well as the relative speed (rate) in getting there.
4. *Social System* – defined as the social units that are involved in working together to achieve a common goal.

In addition to understanding the elements of the process, it is also helpful to define the characteristics of an innovative idea. These influence whether the innovation will be adopted or not by an individual. The first is *relative advantage* – how much better is the innovation compared to the status quo. The second is *compatibility* – how much does the innovation fit with the person's life/lifestyle. The third is *complexity* – highly complex innovations are less likely to be adopted. The fourth is *trialability* – how easy is it to take the innovation for a spin. The fifth characteristic is *observability* – a more visible innovation will elicit greater reactions, both positive and negative.

The adoption process for innovations occurs in five stages:

1. *Knowledge* – the individual's first exposure to the new process.
2. *Persuasion* – the individual seeks more information about the innovation.
3. *Decision* – the individual gives thumbs up or thumbs down.
4. *Implementation* – the individual uses the new process and decides its usefulness.
5. *Confirmation* – the individual decides about using the innovative process on an ongoing basis, and to what extent.

Probably the most useful information for healthcare redesigner is to understand adopter categories, a social systems term. Adopter categories refer to an individual's willingness to try something new. They include *innovators, early adopters, early majority, late majority, and laggards.* The innovator (2.5%) is the first to think of or adopt an innovation, is willing to take risks, and accepts failures as part of the process. The early adopter (13.5%) is second in line to adopt an innovation, is more socially forward, and a little more thoughtful about the adoption choices that he/she makes. The early majority (34%) adopt the innovation more slowly and are rarely leaders in their system. The late majority (34%) are unsure of adoption and usually do so late in the game. Laggards (16%) are change-aversive and adopt very late, or not at all.

These categories have immediate face validity. Each of us knows the extremes very well, from our childhood buddy with eight fingers who always tried valiantly to create a Ray gun in his dad's workshop, to the partner in our physician group who has a four word vocabulary: *maintain the status quo* – the nonadopter's mantra.

Nonadopters will cost you money and drag everyone down with them. You will spend unending resources trying to get them to consider changing, even stepping aside for others. Their owning the process for improvement is out of the question. My experiences in working with nonadopters has led me to suggest the following:

1. If nonadopters are already part of your team, do not spend excessive time trying to convert them. Fire them or ignore them.
2. If you are hiring new staff, seek out individuals with qualities that represent not just your value system, but who also possess the ability to adjust and adapt if need be. As a department leader, I have learned (the hard way) that it is far better to hire someone who has the needed qualities, but needs to be trained in some of the skills, than someone who has the needed skill set, but is unlikely to invest in you, your team, your philosophy, your plans, and your organization. Of course, there are no absolutes – life is full of shades of gray. But if you have your druthers, hire the adopter. You'll save a bundle on omeprazole.

How can you spot the nonadopter? Try the following quote. "The sign of a good doctor isn't being booked months in advance. The sign of a good doctor is being there when your patient needs you." Ask them to explain it, how they might start down that path, and the changes they may consider making. If their response is thoughtful and includes methods that value others, respect systems, and involve change, then hire them or make them part of your Best Practice Team. If they squirm and develop an itchy rash, then give them diphenhydramine and send them on their way.

References

1. McLellan AR, Gallacher SJ, Fraser M, McQuillian C. The fracture liaison service: success of a program for the evaluation and management of patients with osteoporotic fracture. Osteoporos Int. 2003;14(12):1028–34.
2. Rogers EM. Diffusion of innovations. New York: Free Press; 1962.

Chapter 23
Improving Care vs. Transforming Care

Eric D. Newman

Keywords Improving care • Transforming care • Improvement • Metamorphosis • Toyota production systems • Quality • Transformation • Physical event • Behavioral event

The Lizard's Tale (Fig. 23.1).

My apologies for the Chaucerian reference and the double entendre! This brief recount of transformation is the story of Angus. Angus was my son's Australian Bearded Dragon, a fierce appearing spine-laden desert lizard that was as docile as could be, provided you were not a cricket. We raised Angus from a baby no longer than your pinky, to a full-grown 20-inch adult. At about age 3, Angus started to behave oddly. He began scratching and digging in his enclosure for several days, then stopped eating and drinking. We had to force feed him liquids and solids for several weeks. He became clumsy and lethargic. He appeared bloated. We were convinced he was a goner.

We awoke the next morning to discover a wonderful transformation. Angus looked deflated and wrinkly, and was smiling from ear hole to ear hole. In the corner of his cage were 8 slightly oblong yellowish "jelly beans." Angus was actually Angusina, and his/her "illness" was actually being egg-bound. Ouch. Aaaahhhh.

While some would say that he miraculously transformed into she, it was really our thinking about Angus that was transformed. So too is it in health care transformation – a major alteration in physical structure, or thinking, or (preferably) both.

Eric D. Newman

Improvement is defined as making something better, enhancing use, or improving value. Transformation is defined as altering structure, form, appearance, or innate nature. Improvement and transformation are considered in some circumstances to be a continuum – if you improve something enough, you can transform it. A Hollywood example is the Terminator series of movies, where a computer system

E.D. Newman, MD (✉)
Department of Rheumatology, Clinical Innovations, Division of Medicine,
Geisinger Health System, Danville, PA, USA
e-mail: arthman@aol.com

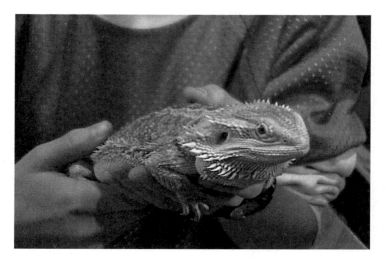

Fig. 23.1 The Lizard's Tale

Table 23.1 Quality improvement vs. transformation

Quality improvement	Transformation
One time training	Continuous education
Many teams with focus on daily operations	Fewer teams with focus on key issues
Emphasis on tools	Emphasis on culture
Work on the obvious	Work on the hidden
Facilitators with QI skills	Change experts with cultural change skills
Aim for numeric goals	Understand changes over time
Reactive response to variation	Proactive response to variation
Quality is a part of the job	Quality is the job

is incrementally improved continuously until a transformational change occurs. The computer system becomes sentient and self-aware. If only Hollywood could.

In many situations, improving more and more does not truly transform the process or the person. Let's compare quality improvement vs. transformation, define each in greater detail, present some examples, and finish where we started – Hollywood.

Balestracci [1] presents a helpful comparison of quality improvement vs. transformation (Table 23.1). His context is a concern that "qualicrats" within organizations may become preoccupied with quality improvement methodology to the exclusion of deeper cultural changes and longer view that lead to transformation. We are not required to agree with all his distinctions to recognize the significant differences between improvement and transformation, that improving harder will not transform, and that we should not sacrifice the latter for the former.

Improving Care

Bataldan and Davidoff [2] define quality improvement in healthcare as "the combined and unceasing efforts of everyone – clinicians, patients and their families, researchers, payers, planners and educators – to make the changes that will lead to better patient outcomes (health), better system performance (care), and better professional development (learning)." Implicit in this statement is that quality improvement needs to become a basic instinct. The idea that we can change things to make them better needs to be imbedded in our daily activities from deciding which morning drive route will get us to our cappuccino quicker, to improving the probability that our husbands will remember to take the trash out on Wednesdays.

Bataldan further proposes that for improvement to occur, five basic systems of knowledge need to be considered. They include:

1. Scientific evidence
2. Care setting
3. Measurement of performance
4. Planning for change
5. Carrying out the planned changes

A key misconception regarding improving quality of care is the idea that lack of improvement stems from a lack of knowledge. This is incorrect. While knowledge is needed, it is by itself insufficient to produce improvement. Most physicians know the right thing to do. They simply don't do it. The same is true of the rest of the care team. Knowing the right thing to do doesn't get it done, unless everyone is engaged and activated in the process.

Examples of improvement in everyday life are not difficult to find; just walk yourself through your average day and pay attention. You have a coffeemaker that effortlessly makes you a single cup of coffee each morning. You drive to work in a car that provides you traction control if you hit a patch of gravel. You arrive at work and (with your single cup of coffee in hand) begin a team huddle to improve the ease of completing the tasks of the day. You wash your hands 20 times an hour using a nicely scented nondrying self-evaporating liquid, strategically stationed every 12 in. You return home to enjoy at 8 pm the 6 pm evening news that was recorded on your DVR. You fall asleep on the memory foam covered mattress that facilitates your sleep, as you dream of the single cup coffee flavor in which you will indulge tomorrow. Everyday improvements are all around us.

It is likewise easy to find improvements in healthcare. Improving access to care by simplifying the scheduling rules. Improving safety by including a time-out before doing a procedure to assure that you have the correct person, the correct side, and the correct site. Improving the outcome of patients with rheumatoid arthritis by earlier intervention with medications that modify the disease course. Improving patient-centered care by seeking information from the patient before the clinic visit in a structured format. Improvements, but not transformations.

Transforming Care

As mentioned earlier, transformation is defined as altering structure, form, appearance, or innate nature. That transformation can be a physical event or a behavioral event is an important concept best illustrated in literature. Die Verwandlung (The Metamorphosis) by Franz Kafka is probably the most striking example of transformation at both levels. This is a story of a salesman, Gregor Samsa, who awakens from a troublesome dream to find that he has been transformed into a rather large .... cockroach. Gregor struggles in his new body to emulate the human tasks he was used to doing – the physical challenge of his transformation. But the greater challenge is the effect on his family. As the sole provider, Gregor's inability to support his family introduces a series of emotional and behavioral dynamics in his parents and his sister. Their behavior and relationship with Gregor undergoes a profound transformation, culminating in removal of his world possessions, reducing his sustenance, and in the end removing him from their thoughts. Gregor then dies. At its conclusion, the reader is left considering that while the physical transformation (human to vermin) is visually striking, the more profound and powerful transformation is clearly behavioral.

Keeping in mind that not all transformation is about changing form, let's explore transformation in healthcare. To be able to transform, one needs a set of tools and rules that will not just facilitate improvement but can help transform. We have previously discussed PDSA methodology for improvement and have also focused on teaming and other constructs that are needed to change or transform.

Olive and Brown [3] focus on the Toyota Production System (TPS) model as a helpful construct for transformation in healthcare. They believe that TPS offers a more person-centered as opposed to tool-centered approach. TPS is more than about reducing waste using "lean" methodology. It also includes a focus on how people can work best together to achieve a common goal. TPS focuses on people and process in lieu of technology and tools. It involves adopting best practice, as defined by that organization. It involves individuals improving their own work areas. It involves creation of a "blame free" environment. It involves everyone developing the skills to recognize what's correct and what's not. It involves visually organizing the local workplace to maximize efficiency.

To achieve this cultural transformation, TPS requires a focus on continuous improvement, just-in-time access, standardization, customer satisfaction, people-centered work, quality, and problem solving:

- Continuous improvement – PDSA, Waste elimination
- Just in Time – smoothing, flows, what is needed when you need it
- Standardization – process standardization to reduce variability
- Customer satisfaction – value in all activities, service excellence
- People-centered work – understanding needs, communication
- Quality – standards, reducing errors
- Problem-solving – root cause analysis, fishbone, understand, and fix it

Table 23.2 Healthcare improvement vs. transformation

Improvement	Transformation
Improving access to new patient evaluation from 60 to 7 days	Providing access to care exactly when needed using multiple modalities (telephone, case review, telemedicine, face to face)
Improving disease control patient-by-patient	Integrated population management to close care gaps
Improving healthcare costs and utilization through rules and regulations	Redesigning payment by incentivizing quality and cost containment

TPS is not the only valid approach, but it does serve to emphasize that transforming healthcare involves people and skills as well as tools. Transformation does not occur by fiat. A governing body "ruling" that significant change will occur, OR ELSE, will likely result in short-term gains (usually through nonsustainable methods such as expense cutting) rather than long-term sustainable transformation. What we need is methodologies and constructs to engage us at a local level.

So we now recognize that transformation can involve both physical and behavioral components. Such transformational events are all around us. The pervasive explosion of smartphones followed by the social networking culture that has evolved around them is a nice example of physical (how we communicate) and behavioral (how we communicate) transformation.

Table 23.2 contrasts improvement and transformational change in healthcare with respect to several important dimensions of care – access, disease control, and costs. Succeeding in healthcare transformation requires strong leadership, a common shared and aligned vision, and a focus on a few key issues.

We have defined and contrasted quality improvement and transformation and have provided examples of each. Transformation can be sweeping, as in transformation of healthcare reimbursement. Transformation can also be personal, as illustrated in Kafka's work. Since we started with a Hollywood example, it is only fitting to end there as well.

The best film example of personal transformation is wonderfully depicted in "Groundhog Day" (Columbia Pictures, 1993). Bill Murray stars as Phil Connors, a self-centered egotistical city-dwelling news reporter, who finds himself stranded overnight in the rural setting of Punxsutawney Pennsylvania during Groundhog Day. Phil believes this to be a meaningless, trivial event whose local pomp and circumstance he is forced to cover and endure.

Upon awakening, Phil finds that Groundhog Day has restarted, and he is forced to relive every little detail over and over, each day starting with Sonny and Cher's "I've Got You Babe" as his wake-up alarm. This becomes his personal Hicksville-Hell. He comes to recognize his flawed personality traits, coping strategies, and emptiness. This forces him to change his perception, rebuild his own reality, and transform himself into someone who cares, delivers, and succeeds. And slowly, the town changes along with him.

In real life, we are not usually given the chance to have a do-over. But we are given the chance to continuously improve. With the right skill sets, and the right partners, we can transform. Improving will get us to the next step. Transforming will get us to a new plane of existence/dimension/level. Scotty, beam me up.

References

1. Balestracci D. Quality improvement of transformation. Sent Monday, August 30, 2010. http://www.aweber.com/archive/davis_book/1YX7G/h/From_Davis_Balestracci_.htm. Accessed 16 Apr 2011.
2. Bataldan PB, Davidoff F. What is "quality improvement" and how can it transform healthcare? Qual Saf Health Care. 2007;16:2–3.
3. Olive M, Brown M. Transforming healthcare organizations for the 21st century. Patient Safety and Quality Healthcare 2009. http://www.psqh.com/novemberdecember-2009/314-toyota-production-system-transforming-healthcare-organizations.html. Accessed 16 Apr 2011.

Chapter 24
Translational Research or Industrial Process Improvement: A False Choice

J. Timothy Harrington

Keywords Translational research • Industrial process improvement • Quality improvement • RCT • Bench to bedside • PDSA • Type I • Type II

> *Scholars in the last half of the 20th century forged our modern commitment to evidence in evaluating clinical practices....*
> *The Crown Prince of methods was the randomized, double blind, prospective, controlled clinical trial – the "RCT" – which stood second to no other method in protecting the scientist and the reader against bias, confounding, and other generators of false conclusion....Broadly framed, much of human learning relies wisely on effective approaches to problem solving, learning, growth, and development that are different from the types of formal science so well explicated and defended by the scions of evidence-based medicine....In the world of clinical care, especially in the quest for improvement of clinical processes, is it plausible that those approaches – the ones we use in everyday life – might have value too, used well and consciously, to help us learn?*
>
> D.M. Berwick [1]

> *The quest must lie in no single field of science. Like a cold trail laid at random across a thousand hills, it must transect with contemptuous abandon all those little patches which the priests of knowledge have labeled, fenced, and preempted as separate "sciences".*
> *Aldo Leopold, founding member, The Wilderness Society in a letter to a friend, 1935*

J.T. Harrington, MD(✉)
Division of Rheumatology, University of Wisconsin School
of Medicine and Public Health, Madison, WI, USA
e-mail: timharrington@charter.net

J.T. Harrington and E.D. Newman (eds.), *Great Health Care: Making It Happen*,
DOI 10.1007/978-1-4614-1198-7_24, © Springer Science+Business Media, LLC 2012

A decade ago, those of us using Plan-Do-Study-Act (PDSA) methods to improve healthcare performance began submitting our findings to medical journals, including many of the examples we have presented in this book. Reviewers commonly rejected them as poorly designed research: "Where's the control group?" Our response was, "It's not bad research; it's good PDSA." We also pointed out that the intention of these projects is to implement good science, not to end-run it [2].

Many academics contend that any change in delivery of patient care must first be validated through formal hypothesis-based research (the RCT), or at least through other large, rigorously designed scientific studies, all within the translational research paradigm. Their expressed concern is that the findings from PDSA projects performed in one clinical environment cannot be generalized to any other clinical environment because of the many complexities and variations across clinical systems. To do so might risk degrading performance, adversely impacting patients, and increasing costs. They wish to subject not only treatments themselves to scientific scrutiny, but also how they may be delivered more dependably in the complex real world of patient care.

We believe instead that both research studies and PDSA projects must be used to their best advantages to achieve high value care, the former to better understand what we should do, and the latter to achieve high performance in doing it. There is plenty of research happening to do the one; we need more PDSA to do the other (Fig. 24.1).

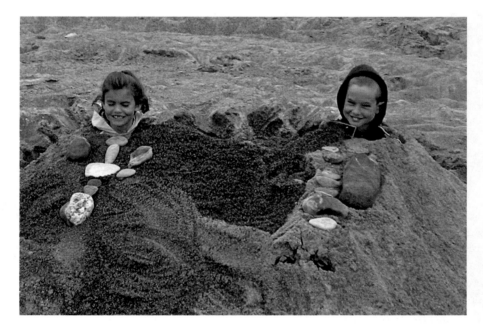

Fig. 24.1 Harrington grandchildren, Kate and Alex Tomes, consider their choices. Beara Peninsula, Ireland, 2004

How Has Translational Research Evolved?

The Institute of Medicine's 2001 Chasm Report called attention to the 17-year average time lag from discovery to deployment of new, valuable discoveries, as we've pointed out several times. Even before this observation, the research community had identified a "bench to bedside" disconnect and had implemented translational research studies to convert basic science discovery into practical therapies and devices – lipid biochemistry to statins, cytokine research to anti-inflammatory drugs, fiber optics to gastroscopes, and on and on.

These efforts did not, however, result in dependable clinical use of these advances, so a second translational research type was added:

1. Type 1, the bench to clinical development piece
2. Type 2, the development to clinical application piece

But the emphasis remained on research methodology. In Type 2 research, a single new aspect of care is introduced into one of two comparable patient groups, while regular care is continued in the other – a controlled trial design. The study duration, measures, patient numbers, and statistical analysis are all predetermined in the protocol. The research might involve how new knowledge is disseminated or how care can be made more dependable, such as physician and patient education methods, nurse coordination of care, or computer prompts to improve providers' adherence to guidelines, among other variables. In any case, the study protocol renders the delivery of care artificial, and the expectation that any one factor will be the magic bullet that creates high performance is unrealistic.

The algorithm shown in Fig. 24.2 of the flow of knowledge from bench to bedside has been widely adopted by the research community to reflect this perspective, but PDSA is missing entirely.

How Should Translational Research and PDSA (aka QI) Be Used?

We view these methods for improving health care to be fundamentally different, but complementary in their potential contributions to improving health care, if each is used to its best advantages. The similarities and differences between translational research and QI were explored in a 2006 "Hastings Center special report: The ethics of using QI methods to improve health care quality and safety" [3]. It points out that the Department of Health and Human Services defines research as "a systematic investigation, including research development, testing and evaluation, designed to develop or contribute to generalizable knowledge." Its regulations view research as a knowledge-seeking enterprise that is independent of routine medical care. Providers exercise their option to engage in research, patients have the right to be fully informed before agreeing to participate or not, and Institutional Review Boards are empowered to protect patients from possible risks, including providers' potential conflicts of interest, when research is conducted in the context of clinical care.

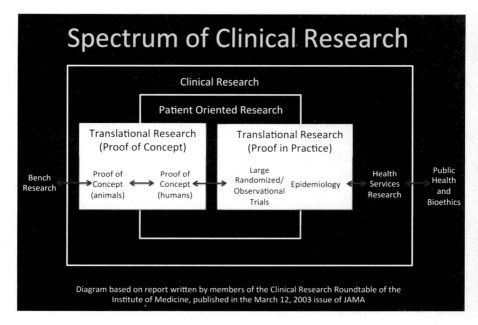

Fig. 24.2 Spectrum of clinical research

In contrast, QI is viewed in the Hastings Report as "an integral part of the ongoing management of the system for delivering clinical care…a natural consequence of health care providers' ethical responsibility to serve the interests of their patients." It includes incorporating research findings into the fabric of patient care at the practice and health system levels. Engaging QI projects and monitoring them should be one aspect of the organization's responsibility for assuring the quality and safety of its patient care, independent from the Institutional Review Board's oversight of research studies. Sharing of successful improvements among healthcare organizations is viewed by this expert panel as important to fulfilling providers' responsibilities to patients and society.

How Have Translational Research and PDSA Performed in Improving What Health Care Is Delivered and How?

Academic medicine is heavily invested in translational research, using large and often expensive RCT methods. This enterprise is well supported by the U.S. Government's research funding establishment and others. Aspiring clinical investigators are being trained in this methodology. The elegance of research study design and data analysis is emphasized. This is a system perfectly designed to achieve the results it gets – grant, then publication, then another grant.

Dr. John Ioannidis, whose own research focuses on bias in medical research, states, "There is an intellectual conflict of interest that pressures researchers to find whatever it is that is most likely to get them funded" [4]. Please don't misunderstand. We are not discounting the importance of well-performed, relevant research; we are concerned about it being defended as an end in and of itself to the exclusion of PDSA.

In fact, translational research has underperformed in redesigning the delivery of care. Nurse coordination of care stands out as the one high impact change documented by controlled trials, whereas studies of other interventions at most show statistical significance in large study populations, but minimal impacts on outcomes and costs. But these studies are lauded as well-performed research, and publications usually end with "More research is needed." It was two such publications in the 2005 *Annals of Internal Medicine* that led David Lawrence to opine in his "Shuffling the Deck Chairs" editorial, "Our goal must be to identify the combination of essential delivery system 'production' factors that can consistently deliver care of greatest value for patients over the lifetime of their illnesses" [5].

PDSA projects are ideally suited to implementing science and improving performance in complex clinical environments, as Dr. Newman covered thoroughly in Part II. They are being used widely in highly integrated health systems to improve processes of care, clinical outcomes, and costs by testing combinations of production processes, as our champions described in Part IV. Support for these projects is generally modest and is seldom available from those sources that support translational research. When performed properly, PDSA work is well defined, but often tests multiple variables sequentially in small, rapid cycle pilot tests of change and before–after comparisons. The size of the difference (effect size) rather than the statistical difference (p value) is the primary measure of improvement. And when the pilots succeed, their findings are deployed.

To refresh our memory:

- We think we have a problem; how can we measure it?
- How do we think we might improve performance?
- What possibilities should we test first?
- Did the changes tested improve performance without creating other problems?
- Can these changes be sustained?
- What were the reasons that some patients did not receive the desired care and outcomes?
- Can we do better yet with further process improvements?

Failed PDSA pilot tests may prove to be as important as successes in informing continuous improvement efforts. (Negative research findings don't often get published). Small PDSA tests of change are designed to minimize risks and adverse consequences, including distraction of providers from their ongoing routine patient care. Multiple cycles completed over relatively short time spans produce rapid change and measures tested during pilots can then be used for ongoing performance monitoring. Practicing physicians gravitate to PDSA because it is a more rigorous version of how they have learned all of their lives, and it works for them in their "real world." It is also fundamentally different that physicians pronouncing, "Starting next Monday, we're going to do it this way instead."

If we accept that all health care is local, then what one system has achieved may provide a quick start for others in addressing similar performance problems, but retesting and adaptation are still required. PDSA methods are ideally suited for this retesting. Dr. Newman provided an example in Chap. 7 of preappointment management being reported from the University of Wisconsin, and then retested and deployed in the Northwestern University rheumatology practice. Dr. Richard Dell also describes the deploying of his osteoporosis program across Kaiser's divisions in Chap. 14. This is the way we will go from "the bench to the bedside to the backyard."

Where Are the True Choices?

The challenge is, or should be, to use both research and PDSA to their best advantages across all health systems. Developing and then deploying new therapies provides one example of their complementary roles. Randomized controlled trials are necessary to document the benefits and adverse effects of new drugs and devices – good so far. The safest and most efficient ways to administer some treatments may require translational research studies. However, the need for uniform study populations in research studies often excludes many of those patients who are managed for the same problem in "real-world" practices. Further, the variables tested, such as drug doses, are of necessity restricted, even though dose-response variability across populations is a well-recognized reality. So once a treatment is FDA-approved, clinicians still need PDSA to integrate it effectively into the care of their more variable patient populations.

How to improve health care cannot be an either–or proposition. This false choice will only be resolved through a broadening of scholarship and teaching within professional schools, postgraduate training programs, and community health systems, as Donald Berwick has suggested [1]. Physicians and other health professionals should be taught the most appropriate uses of both research and PDSA, as will be discussed in Chap. 26. Most physicians become clinicians and will not do research, but will need to be skilled in PDSA to create cultures of continuous improvement. Fortunately for all of us, and especially patients, more physicians in academics and the community are coming to accept the value of PDSA for delivering great health care.

Judgment is required regarding when research is necessary, and when it is time to implement translational research findings with PDSA, or to use PDSA from the get-go to modify and improve the delivery of care. We suggest modifying Fig. 24.1 to show PDSA methods in parallel to Type 2 translational research, as well as to connect it to patient care. The failures to improve care through translational research have actually led some academics to propose Type 3 research. We would ask how many more types have to be devised before someone hollers, "Just kick the ball in the goal!"

References

1. Berwick DM. Broadening the view of evidence-based medicine. Qual Saf Health Care. 2005;14:315–6.
2. Meine CD. Aldo Leopold: His life and work. The University of Wisconsin Press, Madison WI, 1988.
3. Baily MA, Bottrell M, Lynn J, Jennings B. A Hastings Center special report: the ethics of using QI methods to improve health care quality and safety. Hastings Cen:er Report. Jul–Aug 2006.
4. Freedman DH. Lies, damned lies, and medical science. Atlantic, Ncv 2010, 76–82.
5. Lawrence DM. Chronic disease care: rearranging the deck chairs. Ann Intern Med. 2005; 143:458–9.

Chapter 25
The Patient-Centered Medical Home or System-Based Care: Another False Choice

J. Timothy Harrington

Keywords Patient-centered medical home • System-based care • ACGME • Neighbor • Chronic disease management • Integrating systems of care

> The Hatter opened his eyes very wide...; but all he said was, 'Why is a raven like a writing-desk?'
>
> 'Come, we shall have some fun now!' thought Alice. 'I'm glad they've begun asking riddles. – I believe I can guess that,' she added aloud....
>
> 'Have you guessed the riddle yet?' the Hatter said, turning to Alice again.
>
> 'No, I give it up,' Alice replied: 'what's the answer?'
>
> 'I haven't the slightest idea,' said the Hatter.
>
> 'Nor I,' said the March Hare.
>
> Alice sighed wearily. 'I think you might do something better with the time,' she said, 'than waste it in asking riddles that have no answers.'
>
> Excerpt from the Mad Hatter Tea Party, Alice in Wonderland, Lewis Carroll, 1865.

There is no shortage of proposals for mending the broken U.S. health system. Many can be set aside because they favor their advocates more than they solve critical problems for patients and society. Of those remaining, two will be the focus of this discussion, the Patient-centered Medical Home and System-based Health Care. These are generally presented as alternatives, but we suggest instead that improving delivery of care will require implementing the Medical Home in the context of broader system-based redesigns. This dual approach is most important for chronic disease management, the greatest challenge we face, and the subject of our book.

J.T. Harrington, MD (✉)
Division of Rheumatology, University of Wisconsin School
of Medicine and Public Health, Madison, WI, USA
e-mail: timharrington@charter.net

J.T. Harrington and E.D. Newman (eds.), *Great Health Care: Making It Happen*,
DOI 10.1007/978-1-4614-1198-7_25, © Springer Science+Business Media, LLC 2012

In this chapter, I will describe the Medical Home as its advocates have, summarize several lines of evidence that expose its limitations, and suggest how the Medical Home might fit into broader system-based care. It all boils down again to agreeing on

- Which providers will do what for which patients
- How we will make the best use of our current manpower while reshaping it for the future
- How we can coordinate the pieces of our delivery systems to provide seamless, timely patient and population care
- And how we will cut the waste and costs at the same time

None of this will be possible if we stick to simplistic notions such as those that dominate our current political landscape. Neither can we seek to protect our own short-term interests at the expense of others or ignore the longer-term outcomes and costs for patients and society. So buckle up, and let's take a ride into the future as we authors see it.

What Is the Patient-Centered Medical Home, and Why Is It Insufficient as a Stand-Alone Solution?

Patient-Centered Medical Homes are primary care practices redesigned as interdisciplinary healthcare provider teams, including physicians, nurses, educators, pharmacists, and others *that commit to providing and coordinating all care for all patients who are assigned to or choose them* [1, 2]. "All care" includes preventive services, acute and chronic disease management, and end-of-life care. The Medical Home would decide if and when specialists would be involved in individual patient's care.

Support for the Medical Home from health policy leaders and professional organizations is based on the observation that health systems in the U.S. with more primary physicians relative to specialists generally have better disease outcomes and lower costs. The same is true when other countries are compared to the U.S. overall; more primary physicians relative to specialists correlates with better outcomes and costs. This observation also drives proposals for training more primary physicians to provide care that is provided now by specialists, or not at all [3].

Dr. Newman and I first indicated our reservations about the Medical Home regarding chronic disease care and the roles of specialists in July 2010 [4]:

1. Specialists are not included in planning and delivering patient care, other than seeing complex patients or those needing procedures, and only if requested by the Medical Home. This represents no change from the status quo that produces delays and inaccuracies in diagnosis, treatment, and referral for chronic diseases by primary physicians, as our book has documented. Further, it is unrealistic to expect primary physicians and their teammates to have the knowledge and experience to do all of this reliably. Dr. Newman described the present chaotic patient

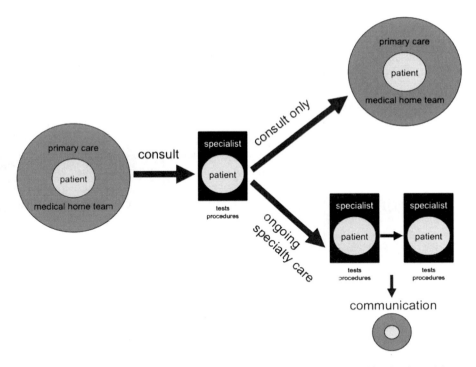

Fig. 25.1 The traditional approach to patient flow and referral decision-making leads to delays, duplications, and unnecessary morbidity. The specialist "waits" to be consulted and independently renders care in a highly individualistic manner. Communication is variable and unidirectional

flow in Chap. 5, and it is illustrated here in Fig. 25.1. This situation is not resolved by Medical Home proposals. As one of my primary colleagues admitted, "We do the best we can."

More recently, The American College of Physicians amended its definition to acknowledge specialists as "neighbors" to the Medical Home, but how this relationship would function is not clear [5]. This position statement goes on to suggest that specialty practices might even serve as Medical Homes for some patients with chronic diseases. In reality, however, patients' needs for specialists vary over time, patients may suffer from more than one long-term condition, and primary physicians actually provide preventive care better than specialists.

2. Early results from Medical Home pilots within Family Medicine have not lived up to proponents' expectations for improving patient outcomes and costs of care, suggesting more complex root causes than can be resolved by Medical Homes alone.

3. Several better-integrated U.S. health systems have established strong Medical Homes without gaining the expected advantages. So they have turned to building system-based disease management programs that include all relevant providers in planning, delivery of care, and continuous improvement projects from the

outset – primary physicians, specialists, and others. Other health systems should not have to rediscover these realities before launching system-based initiatives for chronic disease management.

4. Expanding the U.S. primary physician workforce, as required to implement the Medical Home widely, is an expensive proposition. We also need to recognize that several specialties critical to chronic disease care are as underpowered as primary care, rheumatology being one example [6]. Whether the government and others decide to make the investments needed to expand primary care or not, we need to understand better how care might be delivered more effectively by our existing workforce, and sooner rather than later. And as team care becomes better defined, it may become clear that other professionals – nurse practitioners, nurses, and pharmacists – can provide many services as effectively as physicians, and with fewer years of preparation and lower income expectations.

Why Do We Favor System-Based Care for Chronic Diseases?

The success stories told by our champions in Part IV provide compelling arguments for systems-based care, and theirs are only a few of many. These are the real-life examples of what happens when specialists and primary physicians work together for patients' benefit. Please note, however, that most of these initiatives began with one or more specialist champions bringing their knowledge and passion to bear on transforming care in their own practice while they also reached out to their referring physicians. Ideally, future efforts should involve teams of specialists, primary physicians, and others from the outset, as I will describe below from the Geisinger's experience.

System-based management organizes patient and disease population care proactively across practices and care settings, and over time, rather than through any one specialty, or differently for each patient depending on their physician's specialty more than their problem. It relies on electronic disease registries, robust information technology, disease management programs coordinated by clinical nurse specialists, measuring care processes and disease outcomes, and embracing continuous quality improvement.

Dr. Newman shares the Geisinger Health System's initiatives in this diagram, Opportunities for Creating System-based Care (Fig. 25.2).

The Geisinger is transforming patient flow through their system by identifying the points of care and critical hand-offs, and then optimizing them with broadly constituted stakeholder teams to achieve the highest value for patients. Dr. Newman already introduced this initiative at the end of Chap. 11, and it includes these elements:

• Primary care management is defined proactively, as are the triggers for specialist involvement. These are based on predefined patient population needs for each aspect of care.

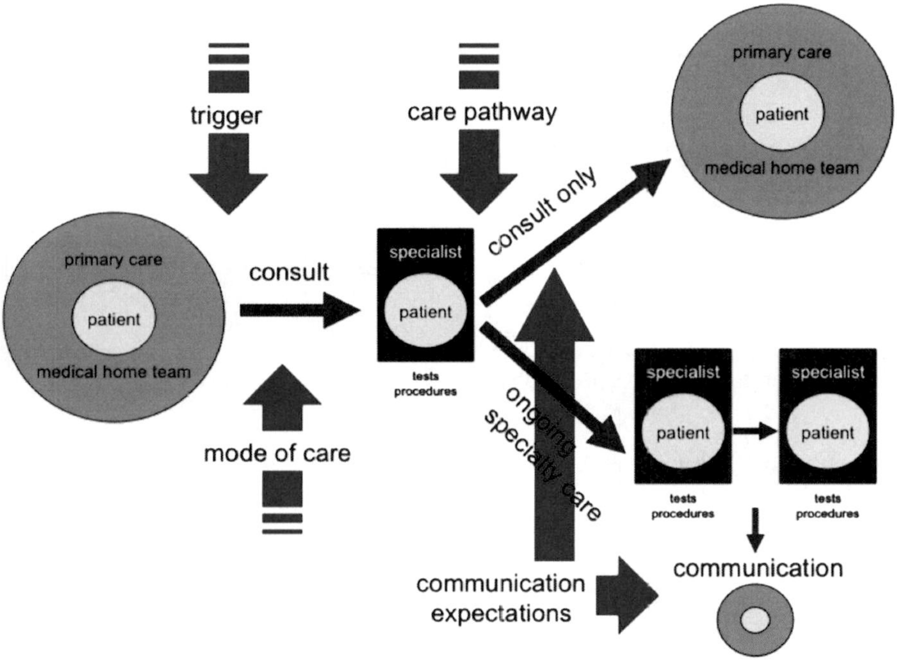

Fig. 25.2 Opportunities for creating system-based care (Geisinger Health System). Focusing on the trigger for care, establishing care pathways, expanding modes of care beyond a face-to-face consult, and establishing communication expectations will allow specialists and the Primary Care Medical Home team to more effectively and efficiently comanage patients with chronic disease

- Care pathways are developed to guide this population management. These include preventive, urgent, acute, chronic, and end-of-life care, based on patients' age, diseases, preferences, and so forth. Specialists may serve as advisors, coproviders, and/or consultants to primary physicians in such programs.
- Clinical nurse specialists are widely used to coordinate patients' care within these defined pathways.
- Alternate modes of care are provided by specialists beyond the face-to-face consult, as is best for optimal care (e.g., chart review, phone call, video-visit).
- Expectations for communication are established in all directions among primary care, specialists, hospitalist, and other providers – and including patients.

Engaging the primary care Medical Home team and the specialists for these purposes will allow consensus building as to what care is optimal, who can best provide it, and how it can best be coordinated. The primary care team functioning within the broader system will then do better what it does best: preventive care, open access, managing patients' stable chronic disease problems, treatment safety monitoring, and advocating for the patient's needs across the system. The specialists will do likewise for chronic disease management and procedures. The hand-offs will be quick and accurate. And let's not forget to involve patients in designing these transformations.

The Cleveland Clinic calls their system-based interdisciplinary care programs "Institutes." They are building them just like Geisinger, and they also have Medical Homes, but recognize that these alone will not provide the integration required to achieve high performance. Similar approaches are flourishing at Mayo Clinic, Scott, and White in Texas, and too many others to name.

How Can System-Based Chronic Disease Management Programs Be Developed?

The requirements have been emphasized throughout our book and are common to all chronic disease programs, including:

1. Visionary physician leadership that acknowledges the present deficiencies, rejects the status quo, embraces change, and supports providers in achieving it
2. Compensation programs that provide incentives for teaming and system improvement more than individual success
3. Consensus among providers to put "Patients First," to quote the Cleveland Clinic again
4. More effective modes of communication among providers and patients
5. Nurse coordinators for chronic disease management programs
6. Alternative delivery processes including telephone follow-up, telemedicine encounters, and electronic consultations
7. A culture of measurement and continuous improvement
8. Shifting from individualism and high process variance to standardization
9. Optimizing patient flow into and throughout the health system
10. Aligning professional training with the system-based care model

With respect to this last requirement, future providers of care need to be prepared differently and present providers need to retool their skills, as Chap. 26 will explore. We need to better define the roles of physicians and nurses for primary care, specialist, and hospitalist practices and customize their preparation for these very different career paths, while also preparing them to work together within teams and systems.

What Are the True Choices?

In summary, we are not advocating for either the Medical Home or System-based Care, but for both, with the Medical Home being integrated into broader, better-defined, and more functional systems of care. The Medical Home should be viewed as one indispensable piece rather than as sufficient for improving health care, and especially for chronic diseases.

This vision offers the prospect of optimizing our present provider work force by redesigning and rightsizing it. It begins with all physicians acknowledging that all facets of health care require improvement, and that we can only do better if we work together. The life history diagrams for atherosclerosis and rheumatoid arthritis in Part I suggest critical roles for both primary care providers and specialists across the chronic disease continuum. The shared priority needs to be helping the system's patients, rather viewing patients as "belonging to" any subset of the system's providers. It's time to roll up our sleeves and work together.

References

1. Patient Centered Primary Care Collaborative. Joint principles of the patient centered medical home. www.pcpcc.net/node/14. Accessed 16 April 2011.
2. Bodenheimer T et al. Confronting the growing burden of chronic disease: can the U.S. health care workforce do the job? Health Aff (Millwood). 2009;28:64–74.
3. AAMC statement on the physician workforce. Association of American Medical Colleges. 2006. https://www.aamc.org/download/55458/data/workforceposition.pdf. Accessed 13 May 2011.
4. Harrington JT, Newman ED. Rheumatology and the patient centered medical home: is it the end of the tunnel or an oncoming train?. The Rheumatologist. 2010;4(7):1, 16–18.
5. American College of Physicians. A position paper: the patient-centered medical home neighbor. The interface of the patient-centered medical home with specialty/subspecialty practices. http://www.acponline.org/advocacy/where_we_stand/medical_home/. Accessed 16 April 2011.
6. Deal CL, Hooker R, Harrington T, et al. The United States rheumatology workforce: supply and demand 2005–2025. Arthritis Rheum. 2007;56(3):722–9.

Chapter 26
Preparing Physicians with Optimal Processes and Process Improvement Skills

J. Timothy Harrington

Keywords Trainees • Process improvement skills • Academic faculty • Shadowing • ACGME

> At the end of our second year in Medical School, our gang of 4 went into an exam room with professor Edwin Albright, and drew straws to see which of us would be the "patient" for his demonstrating a complete physical exam. The "winner" bemoaned the fact that he was ill prepared for the demonstration, exclaiming "of all days I wore my old underwear". We had learned all the pieces one at a time in Physical Diagnosis, but seeing them integrated by a gifted clinician was nothing like we had imagined. Dr. Albright's process became our own physical exam process.
>
> J. Timothy Harrington

> In 1910, in his recommendations for reforming medical education, Abraham Flexner responded to what he deemed to be the "public interest." Now, 100 years later, to respond to the current needs of society, the education of physicians must once again change. In addition to understanding the biological basis of health and disease, and mastering the technical skills for treating individual patients, physicians will need to learn to navigate in and continually improve complex systems in order to improve the health of the patients and communities they serve.
>
> Donald Berwick and Jonathan Finkelstein [1]

J.T. Harrington, MD(✉)
Division of Rheumatology, University of Wisconsin School
of Medicine and Public Health, Madison, WI, USA
e-mail: timharrington@charter.net

J.T. Harrington and E.D. Newman (eds.), *Great Health Care: Making It Happen*, 241
DOI 10.1007/978-1-4614-1198-7_26, © Springer Science+Business Media, LLC 2012

Physicians who deliver great health care need to know

- What to do
- How to do it
- Who should do what
- How to coordinate it
- How to keep getting better at it

Current medical education concentrates on the first skill set – what to do – but not so much on the rest. Being knowledgeable and being effective are equally necessary, and they are not the same. Truly great health care won't be ours unless we work more in teams and systems, get all the stakeholders involved, including patients, and employ clinical improvement (PDSA) methods.

My perspectives and Dr. Newman's on the deficiencies of medical training come not only from being teachers, but also from observing the struggles of our younger colleagues as they enter practice, and those of our contemporaries who cling to traditional habits learned long ago in simpler times.

Physicians need to be prepared better during their medical schooling and postgraduate training for disciplined self-learning during the balance of their careers. The average turnover of medical knowledge is 5 years, so it is not so much what physicians learn initially, but how well they renew their knowledge base, and most importantly, how they access information when they need it. No one can remember as much as physicians need to know each day. Continuing education is also compromised currently by physicians' lack of time and by appropriate concerns about undue industry influence.

A colleague of mine recently asked the techie installing his new office computer, "How come the keys aren't in alphabetical order?" Information technology (IT) is as ubiquitous a tool in today's practice as a stethoscope, yet many older physicians completed medical school before computers existed and have never gotten comfortable with using them. And keyboarding is but a rudimentary first step on the critical path to exploiting all that IT has to offer in helping us to help our patients. Medical information is accessible on the web and on demand (see Chap. 9). Organizing, analyzing, and communicating clinical information ("meaningful use" in current health policy lingo) require high-performing software, and as Megan McArdle put it in an article from *The Atlantic*: "Information technology is on the brink of revolutionizing health care – if physicians will only let it" [2].

How Do Humans Learn to Do Things Better?

The ways humans do things individually and together are generally learned through continuous testing, or PDSA methods, and through teams applying these methods in systems, as Dr. Newman described beautifully in Part II. We also learn by observing highly skilled and more experienced others, "see one, do one, teach one" in physicians' terminology. We did not do a controlled trial when we learned to tie our

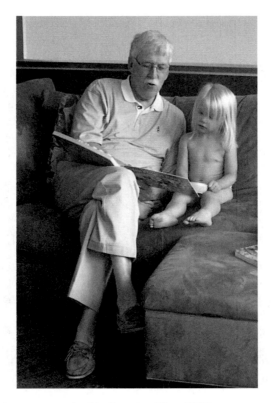

Fig. 26.1 Ursula learns to read with Grandpa Tim, 2008

shoes or ride a bike, to read, or to find the quickest route from home to work that goes by Starbucks. Dr. Newman's daughter and her soccer team did not do research to score goals better; they'd still be studying whether a 3–4 or 4–3 line-up scored more, and since goals are unusual events, the number of games required to adequately power the study would be infinite. They just figured out as a team through coaching, watching older kids, and trial-and-error how to get the ball into the goal!

David Brooks draws upon experimental psychology and neurobiology in his recent best seller, *The Social Animal*, to explore how people learn to do things, and then do them [3]. It turns out that human learning and doing happen in two very different ways, consciously and unconsciously, that our conscious and unconscious minds learn and work differently, and that we tend to underestimate the importance of the unconscious mind in guiding our decisions and behaviors. He explains, "The general rule is that conscious processes are better at solving problems with a few variables or choices, but unconscious processes are better at solving problems with many possibilities and variables. Conscious processes are better at solving problems when the factors are concretely defined. Unconscious processes are better when everything is ambiguous." Our IQs predict success in school, where conscious learning predominates, but do not do so well in predicting our successes in dealing with ambiguity and complexity, our functioning with others in teams and systems, or our getting through a complicated work day. How well our unconscious minds have been programmed through patterning, experience, and repetition is more critical in such circumstances than how many facts we know. Learning knowledge is largely conscious learning; learning processes is largely unconscious learning. Brooks points out that as we learn to drive a car, the process becomes second nature. We no longer see the written page as a sequence of words we either know or not. The routine aspects of delivering patient care need to become second nature, not just for individual physicians, but also collectively for teams. PDSA methods enhance learning and improving these processes.

A flaw in current medical training is that this innate learning is undervalued, and we are not taught how to accomplish it. As a result, we don't develop effective routines, and we don't know how to improve them. We disregard the compelling evidence that we are underperforming. Instead of achieving standardization around best practices, we settle for high variance, waste, and low performance. On the flip side, not knowing what to expect from others compromises everyone's functioning within health systems. My introduction to Chap. 8 provides one example of how clinical process teaching might be provided in medical schools by observation and repetition.

Shuhart and Deming's industrial process improvement methods have revolutionized most industries, and many aspects of health systems. How our hospitals prepare food, order supplies, move patients, and improve safety have all improved. The exceptions are how care is actually delivered to patients and physicians' lack of understanding about process improvement. For example, the journey of "cuisine improvement" started at the Mass General with someone saying, "Who says hospital food has to be terrible?", and then they began testing how to make their food service as good as any restaurant in town and affordable. People from the community actually began coming to the Mass General to enjoy the cuisine.

What Needs to Change in Physicians' Education and Training?

1. A greater emphasis is needed on how we do things as individuals and in teams, and how we do them better. A 2008 paper from the UK described a "preparation for house officer" transition course for new interns. It originally included both didactic lectures about important diseases and therapies and shadowing of more experienced house officers doing their daily work [4]. Such courses have become quite a common way to address the struggles of new postgraduate trainees and the risks to patients during this transition time. In this case, however, trainees were asked a year later to rate the various aspects of their transition course. Shadowing their more experienced colleagues won hands down. Surveyed respondents assigned higher value to seeing how to work than to hearing lectures that rehashed information. They wanted more of the "how to."

When I was interning at the Mass General in the 1960s, many of our attending physicians practiced in the community, but spent their mornings 1 or 2 months a year with the physicians-in-training. At Parkland Hospital in Dallas where I finished my internal medicine training, a community internist replaced our full-time faculty physician each Wednesday. In both instances, we gained valuable insights from observing and being mentored by these experienced practitioners. The favored approach now is for trainees to evaluate patients themselves, and then for faculty to review the trainee's findings and conclusions, "doing and telling" rather than "seeing and doing."

2. Medical school and postgraduate training need to get it right. In 2001, the Accreditation Council for Graduate Medical Education (ACGME) shifted its approach for training program certification away from time- and process-based criteria to fulfillment of core competencies [5]. Programs must now define not only required knowledge, but also skills and attitudes, and then provide educational experiences that prepare their trainees to demonstrate:

   (a) *Patient Care* that is compassionate, appropriate, and effective for the treatment of health problems and the promotion of health
   (b) *Medical Knowledge* about established and evolving biomedical, clinical, and cognate (e.g., epidemiological and social–behavioral) sciences and the application of this knowledge to patient care
   (c) *Practice-Based Learning and Improvement* that involves investigation and evaluation of their own patient care, appraisal and assimilation of scientific evidence, and improvements in patient care
   (d) *Interpersonal and Communication Skills* that result in effective information exchange and teaming with patients, their families, and other health professionals
   (e) *Professionalism*, as manifested through a commitment to carrying out professional responsibilities, adherence to ethical principles, and sensitivity to a diverse patient population
   (f) *Systems-Based Practice*, as manifested by actions that demonstrate an awareness of and responsiveness to the larger context and system of health care and the ability to effectively call on system resources to provide care that is of optimal value

   Competencies (c) and (f), practice-based learning and improvement and system-based practice, were new areas of emphasis 10 years ago. They are essential for the care of chronic diseases, as we have emphasized.

   So what has changed? According to Michael Whitcomb in a 2010 *Annals of Internal Medicine* editorial [6], "In 2006, the American College of Physicians and the Association of Program Directors in Internal Medicine acknowledged that redesign of internal medicine residency training was urgently needed, and offered recommendations for the kinds of changes that should be adopted.... The fundamental purpose...should be...training residents who can provide high-quality care upon entering practice." Five years and several task forces later, this priority is still being studied, and the only consensus is that "a robust faculty development program" is required [7]. These internal medicine trainees are our future primary physicians, specialists, and hospitalists, and yet our specialty's leaders seem to be suggesting that training program faculties are not prepared to provide training in system-based care and PDSA?

3. We suggest finally that the greatest barrier to improving physician training is inaction, as with improving the delivery of health care itself. If physicians need to be better trained to practice better, why not start pilot testing to do this. Let's not stay caught up in researching teaching methods and implementing policies from the top down. Competition among medical and nursing schools to improve programs and trainees' competencies seems important to us. Some senior physicians recall how Western Reserve Medical School shook up medical education in the 1950s by starting students right off in the clinics from day 1 rather than in the third year, and then providing continuous cycles of learning and doing, and learning by doing. Curriculum changes are being tested currently at some medical schools, but not enough. And why don't academics ask community physicians what trainees need to learn to practice effectively. Just kick the ball in the net!

In summary,

- Medical school and postgraduate training should place greater emphasis on clinical process skills. Trainees need to enter clinical practice confident and efficient in their clinical functionality.
- Clinical process skills need to be taken to the next levels, from individuals to practices and systems, over time, and across the various environments in which patient care is delivered.
- Effective teaming needs to become an expectation, not an exception, with clearly defined roles and close cooperation among physicians, midlevel providers, other health professionals, and practice staff. (Perhaps society's finite resources will be better spent educating more nurses, rather than more physicians? What heresy!)
- Training experiences need to happen in highly integrated, effective clinical environments, with programmed IT-based self-learning more than lecturing, and with shadowing of skilled clinicians. Trainees need to see how it is done right. They cannot be left to develop these competencies on their own, or not at all.
- Prospective clinicians must be prepared to participate in continuous practice and system improvement. This career-long imperative applies to information technology capabilities as well. To put it bluntly, learning PDSA methods is as important for prospective clinicians as learning the scientific method is for academic scientists.
- And finally, our current teaching and provider workforces need to be retrained. We cannot accept change by attrition and replacement. This will happen only if government and other payers insist on it, and if the financing of health care is changed to support it.

We have described the requirements and skills for providing great health care in previous sections, and examples of what can happen if these are implemented. Success will require a sea change within medical education and continuing medical education, redesign of the academic clinical teaching environments, and reengaging community physicians in training of their future colleagues.

References

1. Berwick DM, Finkelstein JA. Preparing medical students for the continual improvement of health and health care: Abraham Flexner and the new "public interest". Acad Med. 2010;85:S56–65.
2. McArdle M. Paging Dr. Luddite. *Atlantic*, Dec 2010, 38–42.
3. Brooks D. The social animal. New York, NY: Random House; 2011.
4. Matheson CB, Matheson DJ, Saunders JH, Howarth C. The views of doctors in their first year of medical practice on the lasting impact of a preparation for house officer course they undertook as final year medical students. BMC Med Educ. 2010;10:48. http://www.Biomedcentral.com. Accessed 16 Apr 2011.
5. Accreditation Council for Graduate Medical Education. Outcome Project. http://www.acgme.org/outcome/project/proHome.asp. Accessed 16 Apr 2011.
6. Whitcomb ME. Internal medicine redesign: time to take stock. Ann Intern Med. 2010;153:759–60.
7. Weinberger SE, Pereira AG, Jobst WF, Mechaber AJ, Bronze MS. Alliance for Academic Internal Medicine Education Redesign Task Force II. Competency-based education and training in internal medicine. Ann Intern Med. 2010;153:751–6.

Epilogue: Join with Us

This is not the end. It is not even the beginning of the end. But it is, perhaps, the end of the beginning

> *(Sir Winston Churchill, British Statesman, 1874–1965).*

The quest must lie in no single field of science. Like a cold trail laid at random across a thousand hills, it must transect with contemptuous abandon all those little patches which the priests of knowledge have labeled, fenced, and preempted as separate "sciences"

> *(Aldo Leopold, Professor of Wilderness Management, University of Wisconsin, in a letter to a friend, 1935).*

Now go do that voodoo that you do so well!

> *(Hedley Lamarr (Harvey Korman), Blazing Saddles, 1974).*

Our book explores why health care has reached its sorry state, how we can make it great, and who is already doing that – success stories told by healthcare champions who are living and breathing positive change. We intend the book to be useful to a broad audience: physicians and other providers motivated toward change, patients and the public concerned about its diminished value, the next generation of health care professionals, health administrators and policy-makers, and even for those who enjoy an inspiring read about individuals who have done amazing things. While having a champion skilled in effecting change is a necessary ingredient for success, it is clear to us that the needed skill set is most definitely teachable – to those who are already steeped in the old system, as well as new trainees. And the learning and doing are best done together. The ambitions to share and to teach drove our efforts. They are our Big Hairy Audacious Goals.

J.T. Harrington and E.D. Newman (eds.), *Great Health Care: Making It Happen*,
DOI 10.1007/978-1-4614-1198-7, © Springer Science+Business Media, LLC 2012

What Are the Next Steps?

We need to add what's missing

> I'd have thrashed him to within an inch of his life, but I didn't have a tape measure
>
> *(Groucho Marx, Go West, 1940).*

Start with the basics, and think like a business. Measure. What information do I need to know to run my business? Consider access – do you measure how many consults you get per week? Have you asked how quickly the requestor needs the patient seen? Do you know if you meet or exceed that need, and how often?

Of course, our patients are not commodities like toasters, but it can be clarifying to examine our practices with a business perspective. What if you were running a business that produced toasters instead of clinic visits, and you didn't know how many orders you got, when the orders were due, and whether your customers got their orders on time? You'd fall behind or pay for excess inventory or lose customers thanks to bad service. In any case, you'd be looking at bankruptcy in a matter of weeks.

It simply took us a bit longer to go broke in health care.

We need to simplify

> I made this letter longer than usual because I lack the time to make it short
>
> *(Blaise Pascal, Mathematician, 1623–1662).*

Most of the changes that have occurred in health care are complex workarounds for a failed system. Consider the bureaucracy that has arisen around precertification as a response to providers making low-value decisions. Wouldn't it be better to simply provide a more reliable process for deciding when to order that MRI for back pain? We cannot redesign around the system, we need to redesign the system.

We need to emulate the best

> James Edwards – Why exactly are we here?
> 2nd Lieutenant – Second Lieutenant Jake Jenson. West Point. Graduate with honors. We're here because you are looking for the best of the best of the best, sir!
> James Edwards – (laughs) "Boy, Captain America over here! 'Best of the best of the best, sir … with honors.' Yeah, he's just really excited and he has no clue why we are here"
>
> *(Will Smith, Men in Black, 1997).*

There are plenty of examples of excellence in business. Our business, the business of taking care of human lives, requires excellence in many sectors – service, safety, quality, and efficiency to name a few. So why not take from the best of the best:

- Service from the best of the hotel industry
- Safety from the best of the airline industry
- Quality from the best in the electronics industry
- Efficiency from the best in the auto industry

There are many wheels that are quite round and spinning quite well – let's not reinvent, let's borrow to become "the best of the best of the best."

We need to integrate

True ... there is no "i" in team, but there is a "u" in suck (Anonymous).

We need to redefine our concept of teaming. Teaming is not about me telling the rest of you what to do – the typical physician-led "team" – but rather a group of enlightened providers and co-staff who bring their unique perspectives to the kitchen and work together to serve a masterful entrée. They even change the menu periodically.

Physicians are problem-solvers in our clinical work by nature and training. However, in the case of redesigning our systems of care, we can't do this alone, nor are we entitled to. Much involvement and talent from others is vital for success – other health professionals, managers, health policy, and public health experts – even process engineers from other industries. And our patients and their families must always be at the center of the team. They need to be engaged as our partners, and as our teachers. Remember Dr. Martha Twaddle's eloquent description of patients as our ultimate inspiration in this work we do? "The professors whose gowns open in the back."

We need to be willing to change, and to effect change

Without change there is no innovation, creativity, or incentive for improvement. Those who initiate change will have a better opportunity to manage the change that is inevitable

(William Pollard, Physicist and Priest, 1911–1989).

Knowing is not enough; we must apply. Willing is not enough; we must do

(Johann Wolfgang von Goethe, Writer, Poet and Philosopher, 1749–1832).

Resistance is futile

(The Borg, Star Trek – The Next Generation).

Change is the driving spark to this book. Great Health Care will not result from spontaneous combustion, however: it's really more like a sputtering campfire at high altitudes. We all need to blow on it; to hunker down together in a circle at ground level, patiently and persistently giving it oxygen. And before we can serve as the "oxygen-ators" behind this change, we need to be willing to change ourselves: challenge the way we interact, the way we work, the way we use our knowledge, and most importantly the way we think. Health care as we know it will change regardless. Why not be the ones who change it, rather than being the ones who are forced to change? Be the future.

Closing Thoughts

The teaming concept is a fitting close to our book. We would not be the people we are, or have achieved what we have achieved, were it not for the support we have received from others, colleagues, and family. We are thankful for the contributions to this book from colleagues who truly are the best of the best of the best. We acknowledge that we are only examples of those doing similar great work in improving our health systems, and that we have each been prepared for our work by those who have come before, taught us medicine and improvement science, and mentored us. And we are thankful for our families, who have stood by us, endured our many PDSA cycles, and have shared the labors and the harvest.

We hope this book has interested many, stirred some, and lit a fire under a few. Thanks.

Eric Newman

Timothy Harrington (Fig. Epilog. 1a, b)

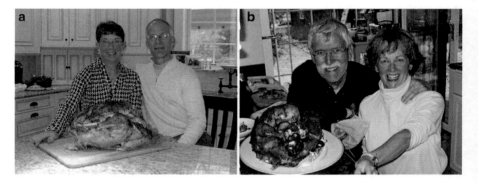

Fig. Epilog. 1 (**a**) Laurie and Eric Newman. (**b**) Tim Harrington and Marnie Schulenburg

Index

Printed by Publishers' Graphics LLC